WHAT YOUR DOCTOR MAY *NOT* TELL YOU ABOUT™
PROSTATE CANCER

The Breakthrough Information
and Treatments That Can Help
Save Your Life

GLENN J. BUBLEY, M.D.
with Winifred Conkling

A Lynn Sonberg Book

WARNER BOOKS

NEW YORK   BOSTON

l be aware that this book may have been
:d" to the publisher. In such case neither
.nt for this "stripped book."

This book is not intended as a substitute for medical advice of physicians. The reader should regularly consult a physician in all matters relating to his or her health, and particularly in respect of any symptoms that may require diagnosis or medical attention.

Warner Books

Time Warner Book Group
1271 Avenue of the Americas, New York, NY 10020
Visit our Web site at www.twbookmark.com.

Printed in the United States of America

First Edition: January 2005
10 9 8 7 6 5 4 3 2 1

Library of Congress Cataloging-in-Publication Data
Bubley, Glenn J.
  What your doctor may not tell you about prostate cancer : the breakthrough information and treatments that can help save your life / Glenn J. Bubley, with Winifred Conkling.
        p. cm.
    "A Lynn Sonberg Book."
    Includes index.
    ISBN 0-446-69080-5
    1. Prostate—Cancer—Popular works. 2. Prostate—Cancer—Alternative treatment—Popular works. I. Conkling, Winifred. II. Title.
    RC280.P7B83 2005
    616.99'463—dc22   2004009581

Cover design by Diane Luger
Book design by Charles A. Sutherland

The author (GJB) wishes to dedicate this book to his patients with prostate cancer for all they have taught him. He also wishes to thank his family, Lynn, Matt, and Janna for their support, encouragement and sense of humor.

Contents

———○○○———

Introduction

For me, fighting prostate cancer is personal. I have not been diagnosed with the disease, and neither has anyone in my immediate family, but I have spent almost every day for the past twenty-five years thinking about prostate cancer and what can be done to prevent or treat it. I have dedicated my professional life to treating men with advanced prostate cancer, men for whom conventional treatments have failed and hope for a cure has started to dwindle.

Over the years, I have seen too many good men die from this disease. I have also seen a growth in the number of men who add years to their lives through the use of new treatments and experimental therapies. By the time I retire, I fully expect that prostate cancer will have become a much more manageable disease, one that can be controlled with regular medication. Some men with the most aggressive forms of the disease may never be "cured" and declared cancer-free, but they may be able to use a number of treatments either currently available or in development to keep the cancer from spreading. In essence, prostate cancer will be stalemated; it will continue to linger in the body, but it will be much less likely to have the power to kill.

This vision of manageable prostate cancer will soon become a reality. Researchers already have quite a few treatments in development that may prove useful, at least for a time. When one therapy fails, doctors have others to try. This approach to disease management requires that both doctors and their patients remain on top of the research about appropriate and effective treatments. This can be a daunting and overwhelming task, but this book can help you make sense of the dizzying array of treatment choices so that you can find the approach that is right for you or the person you love. It will also explain benign prostate problems, which afflict many men as they grow older.

PROSTATE CANCER: EVERY MAN'S DISEASE

A decade ago, most men dismissed prostate cancer as a disease of older men, those in their seventies and beyond. Too often it was not diagnosed until after the cancer had spread to the bones or other organs. Today, prostate cancer is recognized as every man's disease. Due to increased public awareness and improved screening tests, the disease is detected much more often in men in their forties and fifties; and, more important, it is much more often identified at the earliest and most treatable stages.

Consider the grim statistical reality: In the United States, men have an alarmingly high one-in-six lifetime risk of developing prostate cancer, making the disease the most common type of cancer among American men and the second leading cause of cancer death. Each year, about 180,000 American men are diagnosed with prostate cancer, and nearly 32,000 die from the disease. In other words, every three minutes a man is diagnosed with prostate cancer, and every sixteen minutes another man dies from the disease.

What Causes Prostate Cancer?

Prostate cancer is a complex disease with a number of contributing factors. A diet high in fat and low in fruits and vegetables may play a role in causing prostate cancer. (The role of diet is discussed in detail in chapter 10.) High levels of the hormone testosterone may also play a role in younger men; testosterone both stimulates the growth of prostate tissue and jump-starts the growth of cancer cells once the cancer takes hold.

There is a definite familial or genetic component to prostate cancer risk in men of all races. If a close relative (brother or father) has cancer at a young age (under sixty), the genetic link appears stronger than if the same relative develops cancer at age eighty-five. For more information on genetic links, see chapter 11, Brothers and Sons.

Prostate cancer deserves your respect, but for most men the diagnosis is not a death sentence. With proper treatment, prostate cancer can be controlled. Many men have an indolent or less aggressive form of the disease. More than half of newly diagnosed patients respond well to traditional treatments and remain free of prostate cancer for the rest of their lives. Those men whose cancer recurs must face a second round of treatment, but a majority of them respond to follow-up care. And even those men with aggressive cancers that return time and again can make use of a number of new and effective treatments.

We live an era of new hope, and this book can help you take advantage of all the therapies currently available. I support a truly integrative approach to treating prostate cancer, one that takes an impartial and balanced look at the best of both main-stream and experimental treatments. My goal in this book is to provide you with a clear and decisive guide to living with prostate cancer as well as information that will transform more advanced prostate cancer from a fatal condition to a treatable one. Remember also that many people are now engaged in try-ing to make headway in this disease. The future looks bright, so be on the lookout for newer innovations.

NO CLEAR ANSWERS

Prostate cancer can be a confusing cancer to treat. Unlike other tumors, prostate cancer may respond well to several different approaches. As a result, there is no clear answer to the ques-tion: *Which treatment is best for me?* For many of the different stages of prostate cancer, especially low-grade cancer that has not spread beyond the prostate, doctors do not agree on a sin-gle approach to treatment; in other words, there is no uniform standard of care. In these cases, it is up to the patient to work with his doctor to weigh the advantages and disadvantages of each treatment. In later chapters, I will review the preferred standard of care, when it exists, and explain the factors that should be taken into consideration when comparing various approaches to treatment.

As men become more educated about the disease, they tend to focus on the unpleasant side effects to treatment that may lie ahead. For many men, choosing a treatment plan means opting for the trade-offs that they may find easier to tolerate. Anecdotal stories of your best friend's uncle who had a radical prostatectomy and became impotent or your neighbor who had radiation resulting in rectal pain may have no bearing on you and your experience of this cancer.

In my practice, I spend a great deal of time helping men

honestly assess their options and make appropriate choices. Treating prostate cancer can be very time-consuming for doctors, who need to take the time to explain each patient's specific situation to him. A well-informed patient is an empowered patient. He has the knowledge to weigh his options and make informed decisions about his health care.

I also remind my patients with prostate cancer that they need to continue to visit their primary care physician. They need to exercise, to eat right, to check their cholesterol levels, to avoid smoking, to manage their diabetes and other chronic conditions. The chances are good that these other health issues will pose a greater risk to their long-term health than prostate cancer will. Men with prostate cancer need to put money in their 401(k) accounts, they need to plan for their grandchildren's graduation, they need to get on with the rest of their lives. For the majority of men, prostate cancer will be a bump in the road, not the end of the line.

USING THIS BOOK

Whether you have already been diagnosed with prostate cancer or are concerned about preventing it, the information in this book will be of use to you. The overall objective of this book is to turn this confusing disease into a more understandable one, thereby helping men with prostate cancer get through the bewildering process of choosing a treatment program that best meets their needs.

The first part of the book provides a comprehensive explanation of what the prostate is, how it works, and what can go wrong with it. Chapter 1 offers a brief anatomy lesson, describing the function of the prostate and the male reproductive organs. It also covers common prostate problems, including benign prostatic hyperplasia (BPH), prostatitis, and, of course, prostate cancer.

Chapter 2 describes the diagnostic blood test known as the PSA (prostate-specific antigen) test, which changed our understanding of prostate cancer. Partly as a result of this new test, prostate cancer came "out of the closet" as men began to discuss openly their experiences with this disease. In addition, this chapter covers other tests used to identify prostate cancer at its earliest stages.

If a man learns he has prostate cancer, he will be referred to a specialist for treatment. All doctors have biases in treatment; chapter 3 can help you understand your doctor's biases so that you can choose the right physician to manage your treatment. Every doctor will work toward your complete recovery, but you must understand that the experts have honest differences of opinion about how to treat prostate cancer.

As a man progresses through the medical establishment, he will learn about how prostate cancer is staged and graded. Chapter 4 describes the various scores and measurements for prostate cancer. These scores measure the aggressiveness of the cancer, which is an essential factor to consider when choosing among treatment options.

The middle section of the book describes treatment options. Chapter 5 covers traditional treatments; chapter 6 highlights experimental treatments that may not be familiar to some doctors. Experimental treatments are usually available only in clinical trials, which raises the issue, covered in chapter 7, of whether should you participate in one.

This book will help you make treatment decisions every step of the way, but chapter 8 will pull together this information and help you put together your own treatment plan. It will help you assess the likelihood that your cancer has spread elsewhere in your body, and which treatments may be most effective.

The final section of the book covers steps you can take that may help prevent prostate cancer (or its recurrence if you already have the disease) and avoid benign prostate disease. Chapter 9 covers natural remedies, including herbs and nutritional supplements. Chapter 10 describes the potential role of a balanced diet in reducing your cancer risk. Men with close relatives who have had prostate cancer face a greater risk of developing the disease; chapter 11 describes steps your loved ones can take to lower this risk as much as possible.

Finally, it is important to know that millions of men share your situation. Chapter 12 describes how you can find a support group, which can be an outstanding source of information and emotional support for you and for your family members.

BEFORE YOU BEGIN

When making decisions about your medical care, you should openly discuss all matters with your physician or physicians. Use the information here to open dialogue about treatment options and about possible changes in your diet and lifestyle to help prevent cancer. Do not begin using any herbs, nutritional supplements, or other over-the-counter products without informing your supervising physician. Some of these natural remedies can interfere with test results or cause unwanted side effects. Your physician *must* remain fully informed of all steps you are taking to combat this disease and improve your prostate health. The best way to end up with a treatment program that will suit your individual needs is to work *with* your health care provider.

WHAT YOUR DOCTOR
MAY *NOT* TELL YOU
ABOUT™
PROSTATE CANCER

It's Time You Got to Know Your Prostate: Understanding the Organ and What Can Go Wrong with It

Most of my patients—even well-informed men—don't know where their prostate is or what it does. Of course, they are familiar with their external sex organs, such as their testes and penis. They know about semen and ejaculation, but they aren't sure exactly where the ejaculate comes from. The prostate is a neglected organ; men don't usually think about it—and they don't really need to—until something goes wrong.

Unfortunately, many men will someday learn about this "hidden" organ when they experience prostate disease or prostate cancer. Each year, more than 1,000,000 men are diagnosed with a prostate disease, and another 180,000 with prostate cancer.

In general terms, there are three potential prostate problem areas: benign prostatic hyperplasia (BPH), prostatitis, and prostate cancer. In this chapter, I will explain the function of the prostate in the body and review the most common noncancerous problems that can arise. The material in chapters 9, 10, and 11 will help you treat and prevent these conditions. Prostate cancer will be discussed in the remaining chapters.

UNDERSTANDING YOUR PROSTATE

The prostate is a walnut-shaped organ sandwiched between the bladder and the rectum. It performs several functions in the body:

• *The prostate produces most of a man's semen or ejaculate fluid.* Semen consists of sperm (produced in the testes), prostatic fluid (produced in the glandular tissue of the prostate), and seminal vesicle fluid (produced in the seminal vesicles, which are attached to the prostate). Seminal fluid nourishes the sperm and helps it survive and move through the acidic environment in the vagina. As figure 1.1 shows, a tube, known as the vas deferens, joins the prostatic urethra. During orgasm and ejaculation, the sperm passes from the testes to the prostatic urethra, where it mixes with the clear fluid secreted directly into the urethra by the prostate and the seminal vesicle. This mixture then passes through the urethra and out the end of the penis.

• *The prostate helps pump fluid out of the penis.* The prostate switches into gear during the early phase of sexual excitement, before ejaculation takes place. During orgasm, the muscles in the prostate squeeze the fluid out of the glandular tissue and into the urethra; the same muscular contractions pump the fluid mixture out of the penis. (The prostate is about 70 percent glandular tissue and 30 percent fibromuscular tissue.)

• *The prostate helps protect a man's urinary tract from infection.* (The word *prostate* comes from the Greek word for "pro-

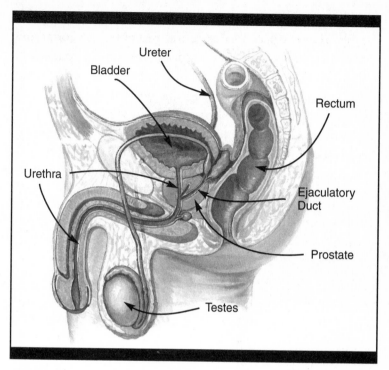

Figure 1.1 As this illustration shows, the prostate (located just below the bladder) is surrounded by a number of other organs and vulnerable structures.

tector.") Prostatic fluid may help neutralize and wash away harmful bacteria that may enter the urethra.

LIFE WITHOUT A PROSTATE

The prostate is an expendable organ; a man can live without it. Surgery to remove part or all of the prostate is sometimes recommended when a man has prostate cancer or certain forms of benign prostate disease described later in this chapter. Because the prostate is surrounded by a number of critical arteries, nerves, and muscles, prostate surgery leaves a man vulnerable to impotence, incontinence, and other complications.

If a man has his prostate removed and remains potent, he will probably experience a reduction in overall semen volume, or "dry ejaculate." In other words, he will feel the sensation of orgasm, but little fluid will be produced. Sperm may be present, but almost never enough to impregnate a woman, although it can happen.

While complications of prostate disease can be significant, most men do not need to face these issues until later in life. From birth until puberty, the prostate grows very little. At puberty, the prostate usually doubles in size, reaching a weight of about one ounce. In most men, the prostate then remains unchanged for the next few decades. After age forty, however, most men experience some degree of prostate growth that can lead to BPH (see below). The more significant problem as men enter this stage of life is not prostate cancer, but other complications.

BENIGN PROSTATIC HYPERPLASIA (BPH)

Benign prostatic hyperplasia (BPH) is so common that it is often considered an inevitable part of growing older. According to estimates by the American Foundation for Urologic Disease, more than half of men age fifty and above have enlarged prostates. The number steadily increases with age; by eighty, about 80 percent of men have prostate enlargement, and many will need treatment.

In simple terms, *BPH* is the medical term for a prostate enlargement that leads to the decreased flow of urine through the prostatic urethra, a tube that passes through the center of the prostate, allowing urine to drain from the bladder out through the penis. Where the urethra connects to the bladder, there is

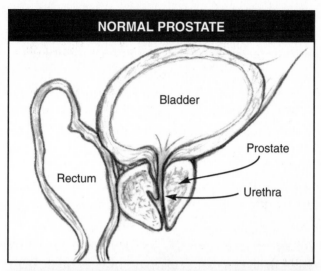

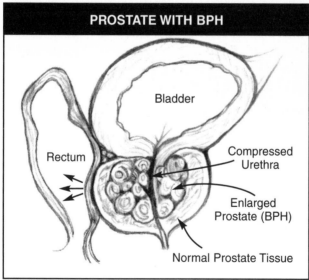

Figure 1.2 These drawings depict a healthy prostate and one with BPH.

an external sphincter—a circular muscle that allows a man to start and stop urinating at will. At another location within the urethra is the internal sphincter, a similar muscle that operates involuntarily to stop semen from flowing back into the bladder during ejaculation. If the central region of the prostate becomes enlarged, it can press against the urethra, blocking the flow of urine. This can cause painful or difficult urination; it causes men to have trouble voiding completely or to feel the frequent need to urinate.

When men detect urinary or prostate problems, most will visit their family doctor or internist first. Based on the severity of the problem, patients might be referred to a urologist. Some physicians base their diagnosis strictly on prostate size, classifying BPH in all men with enlarged prostates (more than forty grams in size). Most physicians, however, use the designation only when a man experiences some degree of functional impairment in the flow of urine, regardless of the size of the gland.

Diagnostic methods include a family medical history, a questionnaire known as the International Prostate Symptom Score sheet, uroflowmetry, ultrasound, residual urine measurement or post-void residue, urodynamic studies, and cystoscopy.

Family and personal medical history. This should include a detailed medical history and a physical exam. It is very important for your doctor to know your entire medical history. For example, an injury to the urethra (from having a catheter inserted into the bladder during a surgical procedure, perhaps) can create a urethral stricture—scar tissue that narrows the urethra—that has nothing to do with the prostate, but can mimic BPH or even very advanced prostate cancer that blocks the urethra. Blood in the urine or pain in the bladder could point to a bladder tumor or kidney stone.

International Prostate Symptom Score questionnaire. You may be asked to score the degree of your symptoms—and how much they bother you—on a questionnaire called the International Prostate Symptom Score (I-PSS) sheet (See Appendix A) The American Urological Association has developed this questionnaire to assess the severity of BPH and to measure treatment outcomes from the various treatments. Each question is answered on a scale that runs from 0 (not present at all) to 5 (always present). The sum of these questions results in a BPH symptom classification of 0 to 7 (mild), 8 to 19 (moderate), or 20 to 35 (severe).

The last question of the questionnaire is perhaps the most important: How much do the symptoms bother you? This is critical because BPH is not life threatening. All of its treatments are directed at relieving symptoms, which means the symptom score will be the main basis for selecting therapy. The big question is up to you: Could you live the rest of your life this way? Are you changing your life? Planning your day around trips to the bathroom? Or fatigued because you have to get up so many times at night to go to the bathroom? If not, you may want to delay treatment.

Uroflowmetry. This test measures the speed of your urinary stream and the amount of urine you pass. It is conducted as you urinate, using a device somewhat like a radar gun used to measure baseball pitchers' throws. To ensure an accurate result, it's important that you urinate at least five or six ounces. This test can identify men whose maximum flow rate is minimally diminished and may not benefit from treatment, or men who have a great deal of resistance to the passage of urine and are very likely to benefit.

Ultrasound. This is a painless imaging technique. It works by creating a picture with high-frequency sound waves, like sonar on a submarine. It can be performed from the outside, through the abdomen, or transrectally, using a wand inserted in the rectum. Though not recommended for most men with BPH, ultrasound may be helpful in diagnosing such problems as obstruction of the kidney, stones, or a hidden tumor in the upper urinary tract; in estimating how well the bladder is emptying; and in determining the size of the prostate.

Residual urine measurement. If you are not emptying your bladder completely, this important test will show you exactly how much urine you're leaving behind. This can be done indirectly, by an ultrasound examination of the lower abdomen immediately after you urinate, or directly, by inserting a small catheter into the bladder and measuring urine quantity after you completely urinate. If you have large amounts of residual urine, your doctor may suggest that you seek treatment to avoid chronic urinary tract infection, improve your quality of life, or avoid damage to your kidneys or bladder.

Urodynamic studies. Your urologist may want to do these studies if there is evidence that the primary problem is with the bladder, not the prostate. Cystometry is a way to measure bladder pressure and function. It's performed by threading a tiny catheter into the penis, through the urethra, and into the bladder to monitor pressure changes as the bladder is filled with water. Pressure-flow studies, using a small catheter, check bladder pressure as you urinate. In these tests, pressures within the bladder are compared to the rate at which urine is flowing. This can determine whether men with high peak urinary flow rates have obstruction. Imagine squeezing water out of a balloon with a small opening; the water will flow if you squeeze hard enough, but generally under high pressure.

Cystoscopy. This test, usually performed in an outpatient setting, is somewhat uncomfortable but usually not painful. A cystoscope is a slender, lighted tube (often flexible) that works like a periscope. It is inserted in the tip of the anesthetized penis, and threaded through the urethra into the bladder; this allows the urologist to see the bladder, prostate, and urethra, and spot anything abnormal, such as a stone, stricture, or enlargement. With cystoscopy, your doctor may also be able to see thickened muscle bands in the bladder. Like rings in a tree trunk, these tell a story—that a condition or bladder obstruction has probably evolved over months or even years. Cystoscopy can also be used to rule out other conditions, such as the presence of a bladder stone or bladder tumor. If your doctor wants to biopsy your prostate or bladder during cystoscopy, it is necessary to have more than local anesthesia. This is called an operative cystoscopy, as opposed to the office cystoscopy, and is performed in an operating room setting.

BPH stems from an enlargement of the prostate, specifically within the area traversed by the prostatic urethra called the transition zone. The enlargement might be the result of an increase in the size of the glandular (epithileal) cells. BPH can also stem from a constriction of the smooth muscle or stromal cells within the transition zone. These two different processes may occur to different degrees in the same patient.

BPH Symptoms

Many men have BPH before experiencing symptoms. In many cases, the bladder muscles will compensate for the restricted urine flow by working harder to push the urine out. (This can cause hypertrophy, or increase in size, of the detrusor muscle in the bladder.) It may be years before the prostate is enlarged enough to create noticeable symptoms.

Common symptoms of BPH include:

- Urinary frequency (an increase in the number of times you urinate that is not caused by excessive drinking or diabetes).
- Urinary urgency (the feeling that you have to pass urine often).
- Nocturia (waking up to urinate one or more times during the night).
- Hesitancy or difficulty in starting urination.
- Decrease in force of the urine stream.
- Incomplete emptying (feeling that there's more urine left in the bladder after you've finished urinating; this symptom is usually caused by actual urinary retention, which occurs because the urine remaining in the bladder toward the end of urination does not have the force necessary to shoot itself through an obstructed urethra).
- Dribbling or trouble shutting off the urine stream.
- A burning or painful sensation during urination.
- Pain during ejaculation.
- Problems achieving erections.

Some men develop severe symptoms before the prostate enlarges significantly, while others fail to show symptoms even when the organ has grown well beyond normal size. If you experience any of the symptoms of prostate disease, visit your doctor. The vast majority of cases involve benign enlargement. In fact, it has often been noted that these symptoms are not typically the result of prostate cancer. It is, however, important you make sure that the retention of urine does not result in urinary tract infections or damage to the bladder muscle.

BPH Causes

No one knows the exact cause of BPH. I suspect that BPH, like so many other medical conditions, is caused not by a single factor but by a combination of triggers working together.

Although higher levels of testosterone can result in prostate enlargement, testosterone level changes have not been noted in patients with BPH compared to unaffected men. Also, levels of testosterone tend to decrease as men age.

Estrogen has been shown to induce BPH in dogs. As men age, testosterone levels decrease but estrogen levels remain the same, so there is an increase in estrogen–androgen ratios. There is some suggestion that estrogens such as estrone and estradiol can result in the growth of prostate stromal cells without the testosterone to balance it out. Incidentally, obesity is associated with higher levels of estrogen in men. This is because fat cells can convert testosterone into estrogen.

Antihistamines can also exacerbate BPH. For this reason, men who may have BPH or other prostate problems may want to consult a physician before taking over-the-counter medications. Antihistamines can make the urinary sphincter less responsive, making it more difficult for a man to empty his bladder. These changes are temporary, but infrequently may be severe enough to cause complete obstruction, necessitating a trip to the emergency room.

Several studies also suggest that BPH may have a hereditary link. One study of men age sixty-four and younger with BPH found that the male relatives of these men were four to six times more likely to require surgical removal of the prostate to treat BPH.

Prevention. Steps you can take to help prevent BPH are discussed in detail in chapters 9, 10, and 11.

BPH Treatments

BPH can be treated using watchful waiting, medication, or surgery:

Watchful waiting. Not every patient with BPH needs treatment. A landmark study published in the *New England Journal of Medicine* in 1995 found that no treatment at all may be the best course of action. The researchers analyzed five studies of the five-year natural history of BPH among men with moderately enlarged prostates. They found that without treatment, approximately 40 percent of the men improved, 45 percent had no change in symptoms, and 15 percent deteriorated. Faced with these findings, doctors realized BPH is a dynamic condition and that watchful waiting should be considered an acceptable approach for many men.

Medication. A number of new drugs have been developed to treat BPH. While medications don't work for every man, they should be tried prior to surgery whenever possible. The two classes of drugs commonly used in the treatment of BPH are alpha blockers and androgen-altering agents.

Alpha blockers are traditionally used for the treatment of high blood pressure; these drugs are believed to relax the sphincter at the base of the bladder so that the urine can flow more freely. A few years ago, alpha blockers were prescribed only for men who had high blood pressure in addition to BPH; today, they are used more widely. Men using these drugs should watch for signs of low blood pressure, including lightheadedness when rising abruptly. This symptom occurs more often in men with normal pressure. The three most commonly prescribed alpha blockers are Flomax, Hytrin, and Cardura.

An agent that alters androgen metabolism is also an approved therapy. In the prostate, an enzyme known as 5-alpha reductase converts testosterone into dihydrotestosterone

(DHT). DHT has been shown to be even more powerful than testosterone at triggering prostate growth. Dutasteride and Proscar (finasteride) suppress an enzyme that converts testosterone to DHT. These 5-alpha reductase inhibitors are approved for the treatment of BPH. They are usually well tolerated, but uncommonly can cause unwanted side effects, including dizziness, heart palpitations, nausea, and blurred vision. They may also cause a decrease in sex drive (in about 6 to 10 percent of men) and impotence (in about 10 percent of men). These drugs will falsely lower PSA values by about 50 percent, so that a doctor should be reminded that a man is taking dutasteride or finasteride when interpreting his PSA level. Proscar also needs to be handled with great care in the home; women of childbearing age should not touch a pill because it can be absorbed through the skin, affecting hormonal balance. Recently, it has been shown that Proscar can prevent prostate cancer in about 25 percent of men. The same study, however, raised a concern that for the men who *were* diagnosed with prostate cancer, the drug was associated with an increase in more aggressive forms of the disease. The reasons for this seeming paradox are not known.

Surgery. When drug therapy fails to reduce symptoms of BPH, surgery may be necessary. There are a number of different procedures, but each, in some way or other, involves removing unwanted prostate tissue. (For information on finding a surgeon, see chapter 3.)

• *TURP (transurethral resection of the prostate).* Though it was established more than fifty years ago, this procedure remains the gold standard of treatment for BPH. During the procedure, a urologist uses an instrument known as a resectoscope to enter the penis through the urethra. The surgeon scrapes away the excess prostatic tissue, easing pressure on the urethra. More than four hundred thousand TURP operations are performed in the United States each year, making it second only to cataract extraction as the most common surgery among men over age sixty-five.

The TURP procedure is not without complications. Approximately 20 to 25 percent of patients have unsatisfactory outcomes, according to a study published in the *Journal of Urology* in 1990. Complications include retrograde ejaculation, a condition in which semen flows into the bladder rather than out of the penis (in 70 to 75 percent of men); impotence (in 5 to 10 percent); temporary postoperative urinary tract infections (5 to 10 percent); and urinary incontinence (2 to 4 percent). In addition, a repeat procedure was required in 15 to 20 percent of men who were followed for ten years or more.

• *TUIP (transurethral incision of the prostate).* This is a modification of the TURP. During this procedure, the urologist enters the urethra with a resectoscope, but rather than cutting the enlarged tissue, the doctor separates the urethra from the prostate, relieving the obstruction within the passage. As with the TURP, the TUIP can cause retrograde ejaculation and other similar side effects. Still, this procedure may be preferable for men whose obstruction is near the bladder neck.

There are a number of newer surgical therapies for BPH. These have been less well investigated than TURP, and consequently physicians are less well acquainted with their side effects and effectiveness. Before embarking on one of these procedures, be sure to find out how familiar the surgeon is with the technique. All of these are to some degree still experimental.

• *TUNA (transurethral needle ablation of the prostate).* During this procedure, needles are inserted into the enlarged prostate tissues through a catheter-like device inserted into the penis. Ultrasound energy is released into the needles, destroying the tissue. This procedure is still considered experimental.

• *TUBD (transurethral balloon dilation).* During this procedure, a balloonlike device is inserted into the urethra and inflated to open the urinary passage. This procedure is usually used on young men who are unwilling to risk the sexual complications of TURP and for older men who may not tolerate a more invasive procedure.

• *TUMT (transurethral microwave thermotherapy).* Heat and laser treatments are also being investigated for the treatment of BPH. The procedure known as TUMT involves delivering bursts of heat energy to swollen prostate tissues.

• *TULIP (transurethral laser-induced prostatectomy) and VLAP (visual laser ablation of the prostate).* These procedures attempt to reduce overgrown prostate tissue using laser probes. In some cases, the side effects of these procedures equal those of TURP.

PROSTATITIS (PROSTATE INFLAMMATION)

Many men have prostatitis without knowing they have it. The term refers to an inflammation of the prostate, caused by organisms, such as *E. coli, Chlamydia trachomatis,* and *Klebsiella.*

Men who engage in unprotected anal intercourse, those with recurring bladder or urinary tract infections, and those who have had invasive procedures to examine their prostates or urinary bladders are at increased risk of developing prostatitis.

There are four basic types of prostatitis: acute bacterial prostatitis, chronic bacterial prostatitis, nonbacterial prostatitis, and prostatodynia.

Acute bacterial prostatitis. This condition may be characterized by fever, chills, pain in the lower back and perineum (the area between the scrotum and anus), frequent and urgent urination, aching muscles, painful joints, and general fatigue. Bacteria can be found in secretions from the prostate and in the urine. This communicable disease is common in young, sexually active men; it responds well to antibiotic treatment.

Chronic bacterial prostatitis. This type of bacterial prostatitis is characterized by recurrent urinary tract infections caused by the same bacteria type each time (usually *E. coli*), despite repeated courses of antibiotic treatment. Recurrence may be due to the fact that antibiotics diffuse poorly into the prostate tissue; for this reason, antibiotic treatment should be extended to four to six weeks, rather than the typical ten days.

Studies have found that men with chronic bacterial prostatitis tend to have low concentrations of zinc in their prostate fluid. Zinc in the prostate fluid acts as a potent antibacterial agent, killing most common pathogens. I recommend that patients with chronic prostatitis take supplemental zinc in addition to their antibiotic regimen. Although this might not be of benefit, there is little downside to moderate supplementation. (For more information on supplements, see chapter 9.)

Nonbacterial prostatitis. This is the most common type of prostatitis. This condition is characterized by high levels of inflammatory cells in the prostate secretions, but no sign of bacterial infection. Symptoms include post-ejaculatory pain, as well as the signs of chronic bacterial prostatitis. The culprit in this condition may be *Chlamydia trachomatis,* which is difficult to culture, or other bacterial agents that have not been identified.

Nonbacterial prostatitis can be difficult to treat. In most cases, a doctor tries antibiotic treatment for two weeks; if the patient responds, treatment is extended for several additional weeks. If a patient does not improve, he can take steps to minimize symptoms. Most men find some relief from sitz baths and prostate massage (to release prostate fluid). The pain may be caused by muscle spasms outside the prostate, such as in the pelvis, lower back, or rectum. In some cases, muscle relaxants help ease tension in the prostate.

Prostatodynia. Men with this condition complain of urinary problems as well as pain in the groin, perineum, testicles, lower back, and penis, although tests reveal normal prostate secretions (no signs of inflammation or bacterial infection). Other tests show spastic dysfunction of the bladder neck and prostatic urethra; these muscle spasms can cause urine to back up into the prostate and ejaculatory duct, causing burning and pain. Some men with this relatively rare condition seem to suffer primarily from muscle tension in the pelvic floor. Prostatodynia is more common in young and middle-age men. Many experts believe this condition may have a psychosocial cause. In many cases, antispasmodic drugs are used to help calm the muscles, and psychological counseling may be recommended.

PROSTATE CANCER

Prostate cancer begins when, for reasons no one fully understands, cancer cells begin to grow inside the ducts of the prostate gland. Prostate cancer is the most common major cancer in men, and after lung cancer it is the leading cause of cancer death in men.

When diagnosed and treated in the early stages, prostate cancer is usually curable. Therefore, there is a great deal of interest in detecting prostate cancer before symptoms appear. The following chapter, The PSA Controversy, describes testing for prostate cancer in detail.

———— ⊖⊖⊖ ————

Chapter 2

The PSA Controversy:
An Overview of Diagnostic Testing

If a man lives long enough, there is a high likelihood he will develop problems with his prostate. Each year, nearly a million men develop urinary complaints that lead to a diagnosis of benign prostate disease, and about 180,000 men learn that they have prostate cancer. Among men with cancer, the overwhelming majority will receive their diagnosis before they have any symptoms at all.

Consider a sixty-year-old patient who visited his doctor every year for a routine checkup. Each year, his doctor performed a number of tests, including a blood test for prostate cancer, known as a PSA test. In past years, the man's PSA level had been 2.0, 2.3, and 2.8. This year, however, the level jumped to 3.8. While this is perhaps not an alarming number when looked at independently—and all of the numbers are below what used to be thought of as the limit of normal

(4.0)—this increase in the patient's relative PSA number indicated that something had changed.

The man's primary care physician referred him to a urologist. No tumors were palpable during a rectal exam, but the urologist appropriately recommended a biopsy anyway. The biopsy revealed cancer in one of six samples taken. If he had not had a PSA test, this patient's cancer may have grown unchecked until it became large enough to be felt during a physical exam, or it may have remained the same size for a number of years.

For the vast majority of men, prostate cancer is curable, providing it does not have poorly differentiated cells, is relatively small and confined to the gland. Most cancers now being diagnosed in the United States are not detectable by physical examination, making the PSA test the most common way to detect prostate cancer.

Why Does a Man's PSA Go Up?

The prostate is filled with tiny glands that churn out prostatic secretions. A network of hundreds of ducts connects the fluid to the urethra, where it is released during sexual activity. It is thought that when the cells that line these ducts lose their typical orientation (as they do when they become cancerous), the cells may actually pump their contents backward into the bloodstream, raising PSA levels and providing a warning that a problem exists within the prostate.

PSA TESTING: THE GOLD STANDARD
FOR DETECTION

PSA—prostate-specific antigen—is a protein produced by both benign and malignant prostate cells. PSA levels can be detected by a simple blood test. PSA levels of 0 to 4 nanograms per liter used to be considered normal. Now, however, many clinicians rely on serial PSA tests to detect PSA "bumps." There are also age-specific norms, so that a PSA level of 3.0 in a man under age fifty is considered high (see below). It is important that if a PSA test is drawn, it be evaluated in the context of a specific patient rather than rigidly adhering to norms.

Several factors can influence PSA levels:

- A man with a larger-than-average prostate may have a higher-than-normal PSA reading, even if his prostate is healthy. This is because PSA in the blood comes from the normal gland as well.
- A man with a smaller-than-average prostate may have a normal PSA reading even if his prostate harbors cancer cells.
- Certain medications (such as finasteride or dutasteride, which are prescription medications, or saw palmetto, an over-the-counter herbal remedy) can lower PSA levels.
- Infections of the prostate may cause PSA levels to rise. These can produce no symptoms, so patients might not be aware of them.
- Stimulation of the prostate (such as during a very vigorous digital rectal exam, a long bike ride), or even sexual activity, may elevate PSA levels.
- Age is associated with an increase in PSA levels; a man might have a PSA reading of 5.5 at seventy, and not have cancer.

Despite these limitations on the effectiveness of the PSA test, it is one of the better tools we have available at this time. Still, there is a great deal of controversy regarding PSA testing. As yet, no study has shown that men screened by this test are more likely to survive prostate cancer than men who are not screened. Furthermore, there is a legitimate concern that testing will lead to unnecessary procedures, including biopsy, surgery, or radiation therapy. Scientists are at work developing better PSA tests.

OTHER PSA MEASUREMENTS

In addition to the traditional PSA measurement, there are three other important PSA measurements: PSA density, percent of free PSA ratio, and PSA velocity. These are follow-up tests to further refine information about a man's prostate after a previous test indicates an abnormal PSA level.

PSA density or PSA index. This test refines the PSA number by taking into account the size of the prostate gland. Healthy prostate glands can range in size from 15 grams (the size of a large grape) to more than 120 grams (the size of a large pear). A man with a large prostate gland may have a higher-than-average PSA level without cancer being present. This is because normal cells in the prostate produce PSA.

Gland size and volume can be calculated by a volume measurement obtained using transrectal ultrasound. Men with larger prostate glands may have higher PSA levels, even if they are perfectly healthy. Likewise, a man with a very small prostate might have a PSA of 3.0 and still be referred for biopsy because that level may be high for a gland that size.

Percent free PSA ratio. This is a blood test to measure the ratio of how much PSA circulates in the blood unbound and how much is bound with blood proteins. If PSA levels are borderline (4.0 to 10.0) and the percent free PSA ratio is low (25 percent or less), then a patient is more likely to have prostate cancer, rather than BPH, which can also cause elevated PSA levels. If the free PSA level is less than 15 percent, the risk of prostate cancer is even greater.

PSA velocity. This is a measurement of how quickly PSA levels rise over time. Two or more PSA tests will be required, typically over the course of several months. The faster the PSA level increases, the greater the likelihood that prostate cancer is present. Often increases of more than 0.6 to 0.8 mg/ml per year warrant further investigation.

In contrast to the controversy regarding PSA screening for cancer, PSA changes are an *excellent* method of monitoring a man's response to cancer treatment. Following treatment, a man's PSA level should drop to zero if his prostate is removed, or less than 1.0 if treated with radiation therapy. If his PSA level begins to increase again, this is a warning that the cancer cells have begun to multiply elsewhere in the body.

A RISE IN PSA TESTING AND THE RISE IN PROSTATE CANCER

Each year, approximately 180,000 American men are diagnosed with prostate cancer and 30,000 to 35,000 die. The number of new cases increased dramatically during the 1990s due at least in part to improved detection as the result of widespread PSA testing. Since the PSA test was introduced, prostate cancer diagnoses rose from 15 to 20 percent of all cancers in men to more than 33 percent. At the same time, a number of public figures began publicly discussing their experience with prostate cancer. Former Senator Bob Dole, Yankee manager Joe Torre, author Michael Korda, retired General Norman Schwarzkopf, and former New York City Mayor Rudolph

Giuliani come to mind, but these men are not alone. According to figures from the American Cancer Society, the number of diagnosed cases of prostate cancer increased from 85,000 in 1985 to today's figure—a dramatic rise in incidence in the past two decades.

Does this mean there is an epidemic of prostate cancer in the United States? No. The main reason these figures have changed is that detection techniques have improved. The prostate-specific antigen test was first approved for general use in 1985 and became widespread in the early 1990s. This analytic procedure is much more sensitive than the older digital rectal exam, which depends on the doctor being able to feel changes in the prostate gland. In addition, before symptoms appear or a man's prostate becomes abnormal on a digital rectal exam, prostate cancer usually must have grown to a significant degree. Fewer cancer cells are needed to cause a rise in PSA values. As a result of this new test and more cases, prostate cancer came out of the closet as men began to discuss openly their experiences with this form of cancer.

The other reason there has been a dramatic increase is that when PSA testing became more widely available, men who had never been tested were screened, and many cases were detected. The second and third time a population is screened, many fewer cases are detected. In fact, in recent years the number of new cases of prostate cancer has been decreasing.

Unfortunately, such an improvement in early detection does not automatically mean that men's health has improved through early diagnosis. It is now known that perhaps 40 percent of all men between the ages of thirty and fifty have precancerous prostate lesions. Yet most cases of clinically active prostate cancer are found only in men age sixty-five and above. Unlike a breast tumor, which may double in size in three months, less than 50 percent of all diagnosed prostate cancers require five years to double in size. This means that prostate cancer is usually among the slowest growing of all cancers. If not for PSA testing, many older men diagnosed with slow-growing disease would have lived out their lives without ever knowing they had cancer.

In many respects, prostate cancer is a disease of aging. Only 19 percent of all prostate cancer deaths occur before the age of seventy, and approximately 42 percent of all prostate-cancer-related deaths occur after eighty. At the advanced ages, competing causes of death are very common. Therefore, the prevention of death from prostate cancer will not necessarily greatly prolong life.

The downside of this ignorance-is-bliss argument is that early detection in younger men may allow for proper and less aggressive treatment. Earlier detection might save at least some of the men who die of prostate cancer each year. In fact, prostate cancer is the most common cause of cancer deaths in men over the age of fifty. But what complicates the argument about the benefit of early detection is that if prostate cancer has more aggressive cells within it (see below) early detection may not prolong life.

WHO SHOULD BE TESTED AND WHEN?

Prostate cancer provides no early warning signs. If you wait to experience symptoms of disease before you seek treatment, your chances of beating the cancer are vastly lower than they would be if you treated the cancer early.

Left unchecked, the cancer will grow within the prostate, often in more than one location. The growth of the tumor within the gland is somewhat unpredictable, although the Gleason pattern is an important determinant. (The Gleason pattern, a measurement of aggressiveness of the cancer, is discussed in the following chapter.) In some cases, the cancer will push out of the prostatic capsule, a thin skin or barrier that separates the prostate and the seminal vesicles. Prostate cancer that protrudes beyond the capsule has a higher likelihood of spreading to the lymph nodes and then to remote parts of the body, at least microscopically. In most cases, the cancer spreads to the lymph nodes and bones. Once the cancer has spread outside the prostate gland, it is more difficult to cure.

Unfortunately, the medical community does not agree on when a man should begin regular PSA screenings and therefore cannot provide definitive recommendations. Some experts argue that a man's likelihood of dying from prostate cancer depends more on the aggressiveness of his cancer than when it is diagnosed. Some men with prostate cancer live for years—or decades—with a very slow-growing form of the disease. It is often said that most men die *with* prostate cancer, rather than *from* prostate cancer.

On the other hand, a minority of prostate cancer patients will develop a more aggressive form of the disease, which quickly spreads outside the prostate. If a man has a more aggressive form of cancer, early detection may not be enough to save his life: The cancer is almost always advanced when detected.

I generally support early testing. My reasoning is that knowledge is power. Still, it is fair to say that PSA testing in its present form has not yet been shown to save lives, and its use definitely leads to more procedures and tests, many of which carry risks and side effects. Men may want to be tested relatively early in life to establish a baseline. Yearly tests after that will provide more confidence to the patient and his doctor regarding his PSA level.

The sixty-year-old man mentioned at the opening of this chapter underwent further testing and treated his cancer at an early stage because he had been having regular PSA tests for years. If he had not done so, his doctor may not have recommended that he visit a urologist with a PSA of only 3.8—a relatively low level, and one that used to be considered normal because it is less than 4.0.

The American Urological Association strongly supports PSA testing starting at age fifty, or forty if a patient has a family history of prostate cancer or is African American. The American Cancer Society used to support this approach, but now takes a less aggressive stance, suggesting instead that a patient discuss the matter with his doctor to assess the risks and benefits of testing. The U.S. Preventive Services Task Force recommends against PSA testing.

My recommendations: At age forty, African American men and men with a family history of prostate cancer should begin to get annual physical exams, including a digital rectal exam, and consider having a PSA blood test at least as a baseline. Other men should consider these same procedures at age fifty. Furthermore, many patients may want to continue to have yearly tests to establish their baseline with more confidence. However, men with PSA tests less than 1.0 may need to be tested only every three to five years.

In the near future, there may be several new screening tests that improve on the current PSA tests. These tests, which are currently in clinical trials, often measure a particular part of the PSA molecule that is more specific for cancer. If successful, these tests may be available to the public by 2005. The goal is to have a better way to distinguish malignant or cancerous PSA readings from benign or noncancerous elevations in PSA levels. We need a better test than PSA alone.

Why Do African American Men Have More Prostate Cancer?

African American men in the United States have the highest rates of prostate cancer in the world. The incidence of prostate cancer is 180.6 per 100,000 among African Americans, seven times the rate among Koreans, the group with the lowest rate. Non-Hispanic whites in the United States have relatively high rates in comparison to other populations around the world, but the rate is about 40 percent less than blacks.

Some research suggests that diets high in fat and red meats increase risk, while a high intake of fruits and vegetables may offer some protection. The typical African American diet may be relatively high in saturated fat. Some speculate that the increase in melanin in darker skin blocks the production of vitamin D, which may prevent the development of prostate cancer. Whatever the reason for the increased risk, African American men face a greater likelihood of developing prostate cancer, so they should be especially conscientious about understanding all the issues regarding screening tests.

OTHER TESTS FOR PROSTATE CANCER

While no prostate cancer screening test is perfect, medical science can identify many cases of prostate cancer early if patients take time for regular physical exams. During an annual physical exam, your doctor should perform several tests to detect prostate cancer.

Digital rectal exam (DRE). The digital rectal exam—also known as the anal-digital rectal examination—allows the doctor to feel or palpate the prostate for signs of a lump or nodule. This test should be part of a complete physical exam done by your primary care physician. Before the widespread use of the PSA test in the early 1990s, more than three out of four prostate cancers were detected through a rectal exam. In contrast, today three out of four cancers are detected by the PSA blood test in patients without DRE abnormalities. Nonetheless, the rectal exam is still an essential part of cancer screening. Some patients have normal PSA scores and tumors that can only be detected by the exam. Consider the digital rectal exam a necessary evil; it takes about a minute and can potentially save your life.

Urinalysis. This laboratory test of a urine sample measures blood, white cells, and protein in the urine. This test provides a lot of good information about your overall health. It is not a primary screening test for prostate cancer, but it can detect hematuria (blood in the urine), which in rare cases is caused by prostate cancer. There are a number of other causes of hematuria, including the more common bladder cancer and kidney stones. This test should be part of your regular physical exam by your primary care physician.

PSA test. This essential test is discussed in detail in an earlier section of this chapter.

Ultrasound. This technique, also referred to as TRUS or TRUS-P (transrectal ultrasound of the prostate), evaluates the condition of the prostate by taking a picture of it. These images of the prostate and surrounding tissues can provide a fairly accurate estimate of the size of the prostate, as well as the presence of any nodules.

Your Cancer Is *Not* Your Fault

Men who do not undergo prostate cancer screening have a tendency to blame themselves for their illness. I had a patient who had his first PSA test at age fifty-six. The results came back at a frightening 40.3; his biopsy found significant and aggressive cancer. These are poor prognostic signs. This patient was distraught that he had not had a PSA test earlier. In truth, it is my strong belief that this man's cancer was of such an aggressive nature that it would have been difficult to detect at an early stage.

The bottom line: Don't blame yourself if you have prostate cancer whether it is advanced or early, aggressive or more indolent. Patients typically look for an explanation of why they became sick. They want to have something or someone to blame so that they can make sense of the illness.

While some environmental factors may increase cancer risk in genetically susceptible men, there is nothing you did to cause this illness. Doctors can't identify clear environmental risk factors that might be modified. After working for almost a quarter century in this field, I still can't make sense of why someone is afflicted with prostate cancer or why it is indolent or aggressive in any one individual. All I can do is encourage men to understand the issues regarding PSA screening, especially if they have a family history or are African American, so that they can detect this illness as early as possible. On the other hand, the problems associated with PSA testing reminds us that none of us has as much control of our life as we would like.

Ultrasound is not a routine part of prostate screening in men with no evidence of prostate disease. It is sometimes useful for exploring the prostate when there is some evidence of possible prostate disease, such as an elevated PSA level or a palpable nodule on a digital rectal exam. Ultrasound is of the most value when a doctor is performing the biopsy procedure and during the placement of radioactive seeds during a cancer treatment known as brachytherapy (discussed in chapter 5). The procedure can be recommended by a general practitioner or a specialist.

TURP. This procedure, discussed in greater detail in the previous chapter, is typically used for the treatment of noncancerous prostate conditions. However, any tissue or so-called chips that are removed are carefully inspected by the pathologist. It is not a primary test for prostate cancer, although prostate cancer can be detected during the test. In fact, prior to PSA testing, this was a major method of prostate cancer detection.

WHEN THERE IS REASON TO SUSPECT A PROBLEM

If any of the tests described above yields abnormal or ambiguous results, your doctor may recommend a biopsy of the prostate tissue. During a biopsy, a small tissue sample is removed from the prostate so that it can be examined under a microscope. A spring-loaded "gun" with a needle about one millimeter wide (the size of the tip of a pen) is inserted into the prostate, and samples or cores are removed so that they can be tested by a pathologist. Biopsies can involve as few as three cores, or twelve or more depending on the inclination of the doctor performing the test. A biopsy is an invasive procedure, but it is the only conclusive means of determining the presence of prostate cancer.

The procedure takes about thirty minutes. The pain tends

more toward discomfort. Not surprisingly, the greater the number of samples taken, the greater the level of overall discomfort reported. Infection is rarely a problem, and most patients are given antibiotics before and after the procedure. Most men notice trace amounts of blood in their urine and ejaculate after a biopsy, because the urethra runs through the prostate and the seminal fluids are produced in the prostate. Very infrequently, the biopsy needle touches the nerves surrounding the prostate, causing *temporary* impotence. The situation reverses itself when the damaged nerve heals, typically in a week or two. Most patients can resume all normal tasks the same or next day. While side effects can be intimidating, they should not discourage you from having the procedure. Doctors recommend biopsies only when they are deemed medically necessary.

If a man has a negative biopsy (meaning no cancer is found), he typically falls into a watchful waiting category. His PSA is carefully monitored. If it continues to rise, the biopsy may be repeated. In approximately 20 percent of patients who have a repeat biopsy, the findings are positive during the retest. A repeat biopsy also might be recommended if a potentially precancerous condition called prostatic intraepithelial neoplasia (PIN) is detected. In this case, there is a greater chance of finding cancer on repeat biopsies. (PIN is also discussed in chapter 4.)

A biopsy provides a great deal of useful information, but it is not a perfect test, either. There is a sampling error; in other words, the needle may miss a cancerous region of the prostate even if disease is present. It is likely that the higher the number of cores taken, the greater the accuracy of the test.

If a man's biopsy indicates that cancer is present, he will be referred to a specialist for cancer treatment. The following chapter explains the types of specialists and questions you should ask when choosing a doctor.

By far the most common prostate cancer diagnosed is adenocarcinoma. There are rare other cancers of the prostate, however, including sarcoma or lymphoma. Also, the prostate can very rarely be directly invaded by another cancer occurring in the pelvis, such as bladder or colon cancer. Also very rarely, the prostate can be the site of a metastatic tumor deposit. This book deals almost exclusively with the most common form of prostate cancer, adenocarcinoma.

Chapter 3

A Critical Decision:
Choosing the Right Doctor

A man must face prostate cancer one step at a time. If he learns he has an abnormal PSA test or his primary care physician detects a nodule during a digital rectal exam, he may be encouraged to see a urologist to have a biopsy to determine if he has cancer and if so, to characterize the type of cancer present. At this point, most men are referred to other specialists for additional testing and treatment.

Some treatment decisions in medicine are easy to make; others can be agonizing. Unfortunately, when you have prostate cancer, selecting a doctor can fall into the latter category because it will seem as if there's a lot riding on your decision. In some cases, the doctor you choose may determine the type of cancer treatment you choose.

Although doctors may not admit it, most physicians are biased in how they treat patients with prostate cancer: They believe their approach is superior to others. Talk to a surgeon and he or she may recommend surgery; talk to a radiation oncologist (a cancer specialist with expertise in radiation) and he or she will often recommend radiation therapy. It is important, however, to be open-minded about treatment options, especially in the treatment of prostate cancer, because there are several approaches that promise good outcomes. It is also important that physicians be aware of their biases, and present them as such when talking to their patients.

To make matters still more confusing, if you are weighing several points of view in attempt to make a decision about your treatment, it may not matter much whose advice you follow. Your chances of long-term survival may be equal regardless of which approach you choose. For early stages of prostate cancer treatment, the medical literature does not categorically show that one treatment is better than another.

In my practice as a medical oncologist, most of the patients I see have advanced cancer. Many of them have previously been treated with surgery and radiation, although their cancer eventually returned. Often patients feel that they made the wrong "choice." But, in my experience, it is unlikely that the recurrence rate will be vastly different among the various treatment options.

Bias on the part of physicians is not wrong. What is more useful to patients, however, is when physicians explain that some of their advice stems from bias. In many cases, the physician's advice might stem from what is considered by most physicians to be "standard of care." These kinds of recommendations are often based on at least two studies demonstrating that one treatment is superior to another in respect to outcome, side effects, or both.

Consider a sixty-three-year-old patient who came to me for advice on how to treat his prostate cancer. His diagnosis of prostate cancer was precipitated as a result of an elevated PSA

(6.5). He had been getting regular PSA tests, and his level had been creeping up for years. Once it reached 6.5, the man's primary care physician referred him to a urologist, a surgeon with expertise in the male reproductive organs. Although the urologist determined that the patient had a normal digital rectal exam (DRE), he appropriately recommended a biopsy. Twelve cores were taken and three were positive for cancer, all on one side.

The urologist recommended a radical prostatectomy. "Surgery is the best option for you," the urologist stated. At sixty-three, the man had years of life ahead of him; he didn't have any heart problems and was in good overall health for an operation.

"Do I have other options?" the patient asked, fearful of impotence and other possible complications of surgery. "You could try radiation, but it's not as good and it has unpleasant side effects," the doctor responded. "Think about it and call me back if you want to book the surgery."

The patient had just received his diagnosis. Although he was bewildered, he felt the need to consider alternative treatments. This physician implied that his decision should not be challenged. This experience is not uncommon: Many doctors don't take the time to discuss other treatment options with their patients or even offer referrals to other physicians who may treat these cancers differently. Making a decision about what the patient perceives as a life-or-death issue is a process, and most men need time and additional information to feel comfortable making an informed choice.

This man sought a second opinion. He visited a radiation oncologist who, not surprisingly, recommended radiation therapy. He was just as dismissive as the surgeon about alternative therapies; neither physician took the time to help the patient understand that there are trade-offs in either course of treatment.

After attending a support group for men with prostate cancer, the man was referred to me. In my practice, I strive to help a patient choose the treatment that is right for him. There are no free rides when it comes to cancer therapy; the patient (and his family) must decide which risks or potential threats to quality of life, both short term and long term, he can tolerate.

This is best accomplished if the patient is fully informed of the possible side effects so that he knows what to expect. A patient's reaction to an expected side effect is very different from his response to something that comes as an unwelcome surprise. We can accept difficult situations when we consciously choose them. In fact, we often find the same situation far more tolerable when we expect it than when it catches us unprepared. For many men, it helps to have the power to choose possible side effects; it is better to have some control over a situation than to feel completely powerless and at the mercy of a threatening disease.

Before making any kind of decision, a man needs to have a thorough understanding of the disease and *all* the treatment options. I try to sit down and talk with the patient and his spouse or partner. I need to know how he feels about the side effects. I need to know how important their sex life is to them. I find that the importance of sex varies greatly, from men whose sexuality is an essential part of their self-image to men who report that the sexual part of their lives was over long before they were diagnosed with the cancer.

Treatment for prostate cancer carries with it very different side effects. Some men are anxious about anesthesia (or they are in poor health and may not tolerate anesthesia very well). Some men work at jobs in which an extended leave of absence during recovery could be a hardship. Some men may have to weigh the cost of various procedures because they have limited health insurance coverage (or no coverage at all).

Many men have a visceral response: They want the cancer out—the sooner, the better. These men do not want to wait six to eight weeks for radiation therapy to shrink the tumors; they want the cancer cut from their bodies so that when they wake from surgery they are theoretically cancer-free. This issue, although seemingly irrational, is very real for some patients, and a reason to choose surgery. A good doctor should help the patient choose the right treatment by considering his physical and mental well-being.

Ultimately, I met with the sixty-three-year-old cancer patient, and we weighed his options and the pros and cons of various treatments. I could not tell him what to do, but I could reassure him that his outcome would very likely be the same regardless of which course of treatment he chose. In the end, he would have to decide which side effects he could best tolerate. When he saw the decision in that light, it was very clear to him what his decision should be.

CHOOSING A SPECIALIST

The first question you must ask yourself is: *Who should my doctor be?* If at all appropriate, I recommend that you meet with a urologist and a radiation oncologist to gather two different points of view about your treatment. The doctor's area of expertise will make more difference than whether he or she is affiliated with a cancer treatment center, private practice, or teaching hospital. Your primary care physician will probably be able to make referrals and help you work within the restraints of your health insurance plan. Ultimately, it will be up to you to consider all of the information you hear and make up your own mind as to which approach seems right for you.

The urologist is a surgeon who specializes in the treatment of the male and female urinary tract and the male reproductive organs. To qualify for certification by the American Board of Urology, a candidate must complete an approved urologic residency program. A minimum of five years of clinical postgraduate education is required, including one year of general surgery, three years of clinical urology, and one year of either general surgery, urology, or another approved discipline. Qualified physicians must also pass a written exam and a second certifying exam. (To confirm a particular physician's credentials, contact the American Board of Urology, 2216 Ivy Road, Suite 210, Charlottesville, VA 22903; 804-979-0059.)

The radiation oncologist specializes in the use of radiation in the treatment of cancer. Some radiation oncologists further specialize in the treatment of prostate cancer. After completing four years of medical school, a radiation oncologist completes a medical (rather than a surgical) internship, followed by four years of training on the physics of delivering internal and external radiation to patients with a wide range of cancers.

QUESTIONS TO ASK YOUR DOCTOR

It is appropriate to interview doctors before choosing the right person to handle your care. While every insurance plan is different, most plans cover one second opinion (you will probably need to have the visit preauthorized by your primary physician for your insurance coverage).

Think about the questions you want to ask and write them down before you go. It is unlikely you will remember them all if you rely on your memory. Consider the following questions for every doctor:

- How many procedures (either surgeries or radiation treatments) have you done? (You want a doctor who has performed at least 150 or 200 procedures.)
- How many procedures have you done in the last month? (You want someone who does eight to ten procedures a month so that he or she has a lot of recent practice.)
- How many of your patients experience complications from the procedure? (There is no way to check the physician's claim, except to know that a doctor who tells you there are never any complications is not being forthright. The same applies to other side effects of treatment.)
- How many of your patients experience impotence after the procedure? How do you define impotence?
- How many of your patients experience incontinence? How do you define *incontinence*—minor leaking or no bladder control at all?
- How long do these side effects usually last?
- How long will I be out of work?
- Will I have any limitations on lifting and movement?
- When will I be able to resume sexual activity?
- What options are there for helping us regain some type of sexual intimacy?
- May I have the names of some of your patients who have had this procedure done recently so I can discuss the experience with them? (Don't expect the doctor to give you the names of the last four patients he or she saw; patients with good outcomes will be chosen. You can still gain useful information if you follow up, however. In addition, your doctor will have to respect the confidentiality of his or her patients; some may not want to discuss their medical history with someone they don't know. In fact, your physician has to seek the permission of his or her patients prior to giving you the names.)

- What kind of follow-up care should I expect?
- Who will be available to answer any questions I might have before or after treatment?
- Do you accept my insurance?

For a urologist or surgeon, you should ask these additional questions:

- When you perform nerve-sparing surgery (described in chapter 5), how often is the procedure a success?
- Am I a candidate for a nerve-sparing procedure? (Patients with aggressive cancers may not be appropriate candidates.)
- How often and when are men able to have erections after surgery?
- If a man is able to have an erection, will it be firm enough for penetration and intercourse?
- Are postsurgical erections natural or dependent on Viagra or other medications?
- What role will residents play in my treatment? (A resident can attend your surgery, but you want to make sure the surgeon is in charge and in control during the surgery, and that he or she personally handles the critical portions of the surgery.)
- How long will the urinary catheter be in place? (One to three weeks is typical; some research suggests that patients who have the catheter in place longer tend to experience lower rates of incontinence.)
- How long will I stay in the hospital?
- At which hospital do you have surgical privileges?

For a radiation oncologist, you should ask these additional questions:

- Do you have any special experience treating men with prostate cancer or are you a general radiation oncologist?
- Would you recommend internal radiation (also known as seed therapy or brachytherapy), external-beam radiation, or both?
- What type of external-beam therapy is available to your hospital?
- Would you recommend a different form of radiation not available in this area if I were willing to travel to a major medical center? (You don't want your treatment options to be limited by the facilities available in your community, if you have the means to travel to another area for treatment.)
- If I receive external-beam radiation, how many treatments would I need? (Most patients require seven to eight weeks of daily treatment, Monday through Friday.)
- If I have a propensity toward diarrhea, is external radiation an appropriate treatment for me? (Probably not.)
- If I am a candidate for internal seed radiation, would I need to stay in the hospital overnight?
- Will the seeds remain in place permanently?
- Following seed therapy, how many of your patients experience swelling around the urethra, requiring the use of a catheter?
- How many seed-therapy patients experience perineal or pelvic pain?
- What form of anesthesia would I need during the procedure for seed therapy?
- Is there any risk of radiation exposure to young children or other people around me if I have seed therapy?
- How long will it take for the radiation to dissipate with internal radiation? (The seeds lose their radioactivity in six to eight weeks, but they are left in place in most cases;

it is not necessary to undergo another surgery to remove them.)

- How long will I have to wait for treatment? (In many areas, a patient may have to wait weeks for treatment because demand exceeds availability. However, this is not usually something to be very concerned about.)
- Do you recommend hormone therapy in conjunction with a form of radiation therapy?

Many patients feel almost unbearable pressure to make a decision about treatment and to make it as quickly as possible. In most cases, however, prostate cancer patients have the luxury of time. You can take a couple of weeks to make a decision, and this additional time is not likely to have an adverse effect on the outcome of your illness.

I must caution you against collecting too many opinions. I have seen patients who have collected six or seven opinions, hoping to get a consensus. There tends to be a point of diminishing returns; after you have visited two or three doctors, additional input may do nothing but confuse you.

Consider how you feel when you talk to a prospective doctor. Do you sense that this is a person you can trust? Do you feel the doctor has taken the time to answer all your questions? Did you feel rushed? Did you feel at ease with the doctor? Did the doctor have a relaxed bedside manner? Despite the highly technical aspects of surgery or radiation therapy, it is my opinion that a good physician can administer often more powerful care by a kind word or taking a few extra minutes to check in with a patient.

You may also want to talk about prospective doctors with other men who have prostate cancer in your community. Prostate cancer support groups can be an excellent source of information about specific doctors and treatments. (For more information about prostate cancer survivor groups, see chapter 12.)

WORKING WITH YOUR DOCTOR

A good relationship between you and your doctor is essential for good care. You must be able to communicate with each other. Although you may get information from several sources (including this book), it's a good idea to choose one doctor to be your main source. This may be the doctor responsible for providing the primary therapy, be it surgery or radiation. This should be the doctor you turn to with your concerns. As has been made clear, there is controversy regarding prostate cancer treatment, and you can't expect physicians to agree on all issues.

Let your doctor know how much you really want to know about your illness. You may want a lot of medical details: Some people feel more in control of what is happening to them when they have all the facts. If this is the case, let your doctor know. Or you may want only the overview. It disturbs some people to be told too many details. They may want simple directions—what pill to take or what their treatment will be and when it will be done. They want to leave the decisions to the doctor. There is no right approach for all patients.

During office visits, especially during the first sessions when you're discussing your diagnosis and treatment options, it is best to have a spouse or trusted friend with you. This can help to decrease tension. Also, even if the doctor is very thorough, you may not hear or remember what is being said. No one can comprehend or take in much information in times of great stress. Instead, we often feel numb. Patients often think of dozens of questions in the late-night hours when it seems the rest of the world is asleep and there is no one to ask.

Don't be shy about taking notes to help you remember what you are told. You may also consider asking the doctor if you can tape record what is said so that you can review it later. If you don't understand a medical term that your doctor mentions, be sure to ask for an explanation. If you don't understand the explanation the first time, be willing to ask a follow-up question to be sure you feel comfortable with the answer.

Between office visits, write down any questions you might have. You may also want to keep written notes on your daily feelings and reactions to help your doctor understand how you are responding to treatments. Make notes and report to your doctor any changes in sleep patterns, bowel habits, headaches, or other physical alterations you notice.

If you feel your doctor is not taking enough time to answer your questions, be willing to address the issue directly. There is nothing wrong with saying, "I need to discuss _____ with you. I know you are busy, so can we schedule a time to talk about it?" Try not to be hostile or accusatory; your doctor will be more receptive to a clear and balanced tone.

Your doctor probably believes he or she is taking all the time you need to answer questions. In fact, an article published in the September 1997 issue of the journal *Urology* reported that almost 100 percent of physicians stated that they always discussed important considerations such as options for no therapy, life expectancy with and without therapy, patient preferences, costs, and changes in sexual function. Only one out of every five patients, however, recalled having similar discussions.

Once you find the right doctor, you will undergo additional tests to measure and assess your prostate cancer. The following chapter will help you understand the staging and grading measurements used to characterize your particular cancer. This information is then used to help you and your doctor choose the best course of treatment for the disease.

Chapter 4

Measuring Bad News:
Prostate Cancer Staging and Grading

When most men first hear the diagnosis of prostate cancer, they imagine the worst. Many ask, "How long do I have left?" While every case is unique, I can assure many men, even most, that the disease will not decrease their life expectancy. Many men will likely die *with* prostate cancer, rather than *from* prostate cancer. This is because prostate cancer is a disease that typically has a long natural history, meaning that it tends to progress slowly in most men. Quite often it takes a decade or more for prostate cancer to progress to the point that a man experiences symptoms at all.

While the majority of men do have indolent or less aggressive cancers, some unfortunate men do develop a much more aggressive and dangerous form of the disease. These cancers tend to grow more quickly and spread more readily. The results of the biopsy are used to characterize the type of cancer present. Two different systems are used to assess the severity of the disease, one to stage the cancer (to measure how far it has spread) and the other to grade the cells (by how aggressive they appear to the pathologist as seen under the microscope).

STAGING

The staging of prostate cancer helps the patient and doctor understand how advanced the cancer might be and determine which course of treatment might be best. Prostate cancer spreads in a fairly predictable pattern. First it grows inside the prostate. It reaches, then penetrates, the prostate wall, also called the capsule. It may also creep into structures connecting to the prostate called the seminal vesicles, ultimately extending in advanced cases into the bladder, the urethra, and the pelvic side walls. The finding of cancer cells in the seminal vesicles or prostatic capsule is important. It is a sign that the cancer has a propensity to spread beyond the environment of the prostate. When doctors speak of "distant metastases" of prostate cancer, they generally mean that it has hitched a ride via the bloodstream to the lymph nodes; the bone marrow (the spine, ribs, or pelvic bones); or, less commonly, the lungs and liver.

There are two staging methods: the Whitmore-Jewett staging classification (developed in 1956) and the more detailed TNM (Tumor, Nodes, Metastases) classification (developed in 1992 by the American Joint Committee on Cancer and the International Union Against Cancer). Both remain in use today.

Stages are further divided into two categories: clinical staging (based on digital rectal exam, X-ray, and bone scan results) and pathological staging (based on removal of the lymph nodes and prostate). Clinical staging can be erroneous, because there is inaccuracy and some subjectivity to the DRE, and the radiographic tests available are imperfect. Pathological staging is a more precise and objective assessment of your condition.

The staging is expressed as a Gleason score, which is an assessment of the cancer's aggressiveness based on an examination of the biopsied tissue itself.

Whitmore-Jewett Stages

Stage A is a clinically undetectable tumor confined to the gland and is an incidental finding during a TURP procedure performed to treat BPH.

A1: Well differentiated with focal involvement.
A2: Moderately or poorly differentiated or involves multiple foci in the gland.
A3: Nonpalpable, a PSA-detected cancer.

Stage B is a tumor confined to the prostate gland.

B1: Single nodule in one lobe of the prostate.
B2: More extensive involvement of one lobe or involvement of both lobes.

Stage C is a tumor clinically localized to the periprostatic area but extending through the prostatic capsule; seminal vesicles may be involved.

C1: Clinical extracapsular extension.
C2: Extracapsular tumor producing bladder outlet or urethral obstruction.

Stage D is metastatic disease.

D0: No radiographic signs of metastasis, but consistently elevated and rising PSA levels.

Dl: Regional lymph nodes only.

D2:   Distant lymph nodes, metastases to bone or visceral organs.

D3:   D2 prostate cancer patients who relapse after hormone therapy (discussed in chapter 5); this is often called hormone-refractory disease.

TNM Stages

Primary Tumor (T)

TX: Primary tumor cannot be assessed.

T0:   No evidence of primary tumor.

T1:   Clinically nonapparent tumor not palpable or visible by imaging:

T1a: Tumor found in 5 percent of tissue or less of a prostate tissue sample from TURP sample.

T1b: Tumor found in more than 5 percent of a prostate tissue sample from TURP sample.

T1c: Tumor identified by needle biopsy (because of elevated PSA), equivalent to A3 in the Whitmore-Jewett system. (This is the most frequent stage of prostate cancer diagnosed in the United States.)

T2:   Tumor confined within the prostate; the tumor is large enough to be felt during a digital rectal exam, but the patient does not experience symptoms:

T2a: Tumor involves less than half of one lobe of the prostate.

T2b: Tumor involves more than half of one lobe, but not both lobes.

T2c: Tumor involves both lobes.

T3:   Tumor spreads beyond the prostate into the surrounding tissue; the seminal vesicles may be involved:

T3a: The tumor has spread outside the prostate capsule on one side; this is sometimes called unilateral extracapsular extension.

T3b: The tumor has spread outside the prostate capsule on both sides; this is sometimes called bilateral extracapsular extension.

T3c: The tumor has spread into one or both of the seminal vesicles.

T4: Tumor is within the pelvic regions but may have spread to other areas:

T4a: The tumor has invaded one or more of the following areas: the bladder neck, the external sphincter (which controls the flow of urine), or the rectum.

T4b: The tumor has spread beyond the prostate and now involves the levator muscles (those that help raise and lower the prostate); the tumor may also be attached to the pelvic wall.

Regional Lymph Nodes (N)
This is a measure of lymph node involvement.

NX: Regional lymph nodes cannot be assessed.

N0: The cancer has not spread to the regional lymph nodes.

N1: Prostate cancer cells are found in a single lymph node in the pelvic area and are two centimeters (about three-quarters of an inch) or less in size.

N2: Prostate cancer cells are found in a single lymph node in the pelvic area and are more than two centimeters but less than five centimeters (about two inches) in size. Stage N2 is also used to describe prostate cancer

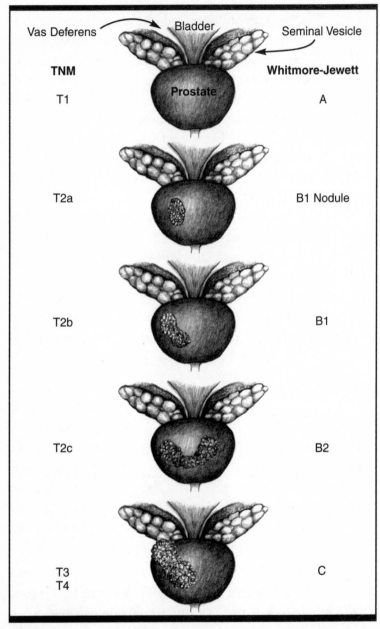

Figure 4.1 These drawings represent the stages of prostate cancer, illustrating both the TNM and the Whitmore-Jewett staging systems.

found in more than one lymph node, as long as the affected nodes are less than five centimeters in size.

N3: Prostate cancer cells are found in lymph nodes and are larger than five centimeters in size.

Distant Metastases (M)

MX: Presence of distant metastases cannot be assessed.

M0: No distant metastases; the cancer has not spread to distant parts of the body.

M1: Distant metastases; the cancer has spread beyond the pelvic area to other parts of the body:
M1a: Nonregional lymph node(s) involvement.
M1b: Bone(s) involvement.
M1c: Other site(s).

Five-Year Prostate Cancer Survival Rates According to Stage

Once a man has been assigned a stage, he wants to know what that number has to do with his long-term survival. No doctor can predict the future, but data collected on thousands of prostate cancer patients give us a good idea of how a man's cancer stage may affect his life expectancy. The following list is based on statistical averages. You should discuss your personal situation with your physician. It is important to understand also that more important than the stage of the disease is the Gleason grade. Both stage and grade are important in predicting survival.

Stage A1

- The tumor is localized to an area in size less than 5 percent of the prostate.

- Almost all men will survive this stage with or without treatment.

Stage A2

- The tumor occupies a larger area of the prostate.
- 70 to 80 percent survive five years.

Stage A3

- This is the most common clinical stage. This is equivalent to stage T1c in the TNM staging system.
- 90 percent will survive five years, but this is extremely variable depending on Gleason grade.

Stage B1

- The tumor is limited to one lobe of the prostate.
- 75 percent survive five years.

Stage B2

- The tumor penetrates more than one lobe.
- 60 percent survive five years.

Stage C1

- The tumor has spread beyond the prostate.
- 50 to 55 percent survive five years.

Stage C2

- The tumor has spread beyond the prostate and also involves nearby tissues.
- 40 to 45 percent survive five years.

Stage D1

- Cancer cells are found in the lymph nodes.
- 40 percent survive five years.

Stage D2

- In addition to the lymph nodes, the cancer has spread to distant organs, usually the bone marrow.
- Less than 35 percent survive five years.

A note about these survival estimates. First, these estimates are necessarily based on older studies; survival takes a long time to measure. There is also good news in that there is a clear trend toward a decrease in mortality from prostate cancer, definitely affecting these stage-specific estimates of mortality. Clinical staging of stage C and D disease is very inaccurate. Finally, these survival estimates are affected by Gleason grading, discussed below.

GRADING: USING THE GLEASON SCORE

As mentioned earlier, the Gleason score is an assessment of the aggressiveness of the cancer. If cancer cells are found during a biopsy, then a pathologist examines the cells under a microscope. A Gleason score—named for Donald F. Gleason, a pathologist for the Veterans Administration who developed the testing system—has been designed to assess the aggressiveness of the cancer cells.

The Gleason score (or grade) is assigned on the pattern of gland formation and the shape of the cells. If the individual cancer cells and cancerous prostate gland closely resemble healthy cells and a normal gland, they are considered well differentiated. These cells are evenly spaced and form a compact

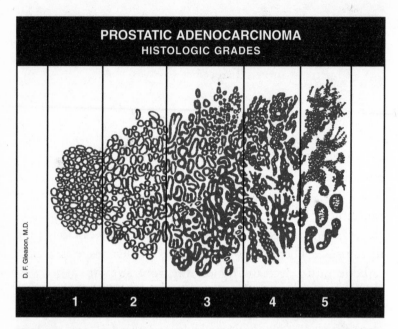

Figure 4.2 The Gleason system scores prostate cancer cells based on their appearance. Prostate cancer cells range in appearance from well differentiated nearly normal cells (pattern 1) to very poorly differentiated most abnormal (pattern 5). To calculate the score, pathologists add the score of the most common cell pattern with the second most common pattern to assess the aggressiveness of the cancer. In some cases, oncologists look at both the total score and the order of its two components. For example, two men may have Gleason scores of 7, but one man may have a 4 + 3 = 7 (more aggressive) and another may have a 3 + 4 = 7 (somewhat less aggressive).

mass with a defined margin between the tumor and the healthy tissue areas. This is a grade of 2; although the scoring system technically goes from 1 to 5, grade 1 is so close to normal that in reality it does not exist. Grade 2 is also much less commonly diagnosed from core biopsies; it is more common from TURP specimens. Grade 3 is the most common grade. The glands in this stage are smaller than normal glands. In grade 4, the cancer glands almost fuse together. As the gland shape breaks apart and single cancer cells progressively invade the surrounding tissue, the score increases to a maximum of 5, at which point there is no resemblance to the normal prostate gland pattern.

As the pathologist views the sample of cells, he or she identifies the two most common cell patterns as the primary and secondary patterns. The scores of these two patterns are added together to yield the Gleason score or Gleason sum. The lowest (and safest) score is 2 + 1 = 3 or 2 + 2 = 4; and the highest is 5 + 5 = 10. Scores of 4 to 6 describe a well-differentiated cancer. A score of 7 represents moderate differentiation, and scores of 8 to 10 represent poorly differentiated cancer. As the score rises, the prognosis worsens, independent of stage.

Fewer than 2 percent of men who have a needle biopsy have a Gleason score of 2, 3, or 4. Gleason scores of 8, 9, and 10 occur in about 8 percent of biopsies. That means that 90 percent of all men with biopsies have a Gleason of 5, 6, or 7. In fact, for Gleason scores of 7, it is often useful to depict the patterns as 3 + 4 or 4 + 3, because there is useful prognostic information in this distinction. A Gleason pattern of 3 + 4 portends a better prognosis than a Gleason pattern of 4 + 3.

Gleason scores are not assigned when a biopsy is negative, meaning that no cancer is seen. Another possibility is an "atypical" finding or atypical glandular focus, meaning that the cells can't be called cancerous, but the area is not completely normal either. In this case, you might want to have another pathologist review the slides for a second opinion.

Another possibility is discovery of prostatic intraepithelial neoplasia (PIN), which may be precancerous. PIN may indicate a propensity to develop cancer in that region or another location within the gland. If PIN is detected, or if an atypical glandular focus is diagnosed, you might be asked to consider a repeat biopsy in six months to one year.

Once you learn the stage and grade of your prostate cancer, you will want to work with your physician to choose a treatment plan for your disease. If you are interested in more detailed information about what your clinical stage and Gleason score mean in combination with your PSA levels, see the Partin tables in Appendix B. The following chapter will describe the traditional treatments for prostate cancer.

Chapter 5

What Most Doctors Will Tell You: Traditional Treatments for Prostate Cancer

When a man is first diagnosed with prostate cancer, he looks for a simple answer to a basic question: *What is the best primary treatment for me?* When men ask me that question, I wish I could come up with a simple and straightforward response, but there are no easy answers, no one-size-fits-all prescription for the care for prostate cancer.

Unlike most other cancers, some early-stage prostate cancers require no treatment other than watchful waiting to monitor how the disease progresses. (This option will be discussed in more detail later.) For those men who do seek treatment, choosing an approach can be difficult. With most types of cancer, one treatment is clearly preferable to another; with prostate cancer, the data are often ambiguous when it comes to which approach is most appropriate for primary treatment. In other words, it's not clear that a man's long-term survival is not likely to be changed regardless of which treatment option he chooses, assuming he chooses some form of therapy.

Prostate cancer treatment can be divided into two categories: primary therapy (the first course of treatment) and salvage therapy (for men whose cancer recurs). In addition, treatments can be divided into traditional (widely used by the medical community) and experimental or investigational therapies (which are in the research phases and have not been confirmed as safe and effective). While many experimental treatments hold promise for men who suffer from recurring cancers, in my firm opinion men should examine traditional treatments first.

PRIMARY THERAPY

Traditional treatments for primary therapy include watchful waiting (careful observation without treatment), surgery (radical prostatectomy), radiation therapy (external and/or brachytherapy), or radiation therapy combined with hormonal treatment. Each approach to treatment comes with its own set of risks and side effects, which will be discussed in this chapter. (Experimental treatments will be discussed in chapter 6.)

Most patients I have seen feel the weight of the world on their shoulders when deciding on a course of treatment. In my opinion, the biology of the cancer is more important than the type of treatment a man chooses. In other words, a man's prognosis is more influenced by his Gleason score, the stage of his tumor, and other factors not identified yet.

Consider all of the treatment options, and discuss them with your doctor. You need to individualize your treatment, taking into consideration your overall health, your age, and how well you believe you will tolerate certain side effects of treatment. And remember that your decision is unlikely to affect the ultimate outcome of the disease.

Watchful Waiting

Infrequently, after a biopsy has confirmed the diagnosis, doctors may recommend that a patient with prostate cancer forgo immediate primary therapy and try to monitor the progress of his disease. This approach, referred to as watchful waiting, involves attempts to monitor the cancer, watching for signs of progression, including rising PSA levels, changes in the digital rectal exams, and often repeat biopsies. None of these methods is foolproof, however, and the disease may progress without changes in PSA, DRE, or even biopsies. Primary therapy—surgery and radiation—often is not started until there is evidence that the cancer is advancing. In fact, some physicians call watchful waiting, especially in younger patients, deferred therapy.

During the waiting period, no one expects the cancer to go into remission. Instead, the physician and patient are gambling that the disease will advance so slowly that it will not threaten the man's overall health for years to come. A man can avail himself of a primary therapy anytime he and his doctor deem it necessary, hoping on one level that primary therapy might never be necessary. At least a patient might avoid the complications of surgery and radiation by delaying the procedures as long as possible. This is an example of medicine as art; the physician must balance the likelihood of the treatment affecting the outcome of the disease against the likelihood that the treatment will compromise a patient's quality of life without prolonging his life. Watchful waiting is relatively popular in Sweden, though it is less popular in the United States.

Who should consider watchful waiting? Watchful waiting may be appropriate for men who are more than seventy years of age, and those with a coexisting illness that is likely to limit their life span (such as advanced cardiovascular disease, diabetes, or emphysema). The decision weighs the risk of progression of the disease against the possibility of death from old age or other competing illnesses. Obviously, this approach is more appropriate for patients with less aggressive tumors (Gleason sum 6) that can be expected to progress more slowly. The appropriate candidates for watchful waiting are men for whom radical intervention such as surgery or radiation will probably not prolong life, while the side effects could significantly diminish quality of life.

PSA density is sometimes used when assessing candidates for watchful waiting. One study suggested that the optimal patient should have a PSA density equal to or less than 0.1. PSA density is calculated by determining the ratio of PSA to prostate size. For example, if a man's PSA was 5 and his prostate was 50 grams, his PSA density would be 0.1. (PSA density is described in greater detail in chapter 2.)

Who should avoid watchful waiting? Watchful waiting typically is not recommended for relatively healthy men under age seventy-five. Younger men can be expected to live longer, so the cancer would have more time to pose a threat. It is often not recommended for intermediate grade cancer, in which the cancer is likely to progress if untreated.

Advantages of watchful waiting. You will not experience any immediate side effects from primary therapy.

Disadvantages of watchful waiting. The cancer may have an opportunity to advance or spread. The major problem with watchful waiting is that doctors don't know how or what to "watch." The technology for imaging prostate cancer within the prostate is still evolving. Without a good method of assessing whether or not a cancer is getting bigger, it is hard to adopt this option, especially for men likely to have a relatively long period of being at risk (if they are less than seventy years old and in good health). Some men opt to be re-biopsied at regular intervals (every year to two years), but as previously discussed, biopsies are an imperfect tool. In other words, some cancers slip by undetected due to sampling error. Furthermore, in many men the PSA measurement in their blood does not accurately reflect how much cancer is in their gland. Therefore, serial PSA measurements will be inaccurate.

Surgery

Surgical removal of the prostate (radical prostatectomy) has been the standard therapy for localized prostate cancer in the United States. During this procedure, the entire prostate is removed and the bladder is reconnected to the urethra.

Radical prostatectomy is usually performed to remove early-stage prostate cancer before it can spread to other parts of the body. In cases when a man has a high PSA or high Gleason score, some doctors will begin the surgery with a biopsy of the pelvic lymph nodes to make sure the cancer has not spread. The lymph nodes are removed and placed in liquid nitrogen to freeze them; they can then be sliced immediately into microscopic layers and examined under a microscope. During the twenty or thirty minutes of the test, the operation is suspended. If cancer is not detected in the lymph nodes, the operation continues; if the cancer has spread beyond the prostate to the lymph nodes, many surgeons will cancel the operation. When the surgery is halted, it is to avoid complications. Others will remove the prostate and all the cancer possible, hoping that the surgery might still be curative.

Your doctor may not tell you that there is a possibility that your operation will be aborted because of lymph node involvement. It is essential that a man understand that he may awaken with his prostate removed and his potency threatened—but he may also find his prostate intact and a grimmer prognosis for his future. Fortunately, this is not a common occurrence anymore, perhaps because PSA testing has allowed for the detection of most cancers before they spread to the lymph nodes. Still, it is wise for patients to openly discuss the specifics of the planned operation with their doctor before surgery.

The operation lasts about two to four hours. Men who undergo radical prostatectomy should expect to spend at least two to four days in the hospital; full recovery takes three to six months. Because of short hospital stays, most men leave the hospital with a urinary catheter in place and prescriptions for oral narcotics. (The catheter is usually removed within the first weeks.) The rule of thumb is that once a man can walk, eat solid food, and control pain with oral medication, he is discharged. Many patients receive some care from visiting nurses.

In rare cases, hormonal therapy is used before surgery in men with more aggressive cancers. (Hormone therapy is discussed later in this chapter.) Researchers have found that men who have hormone therapy prior to surgery often have clearer margins or edges around their tumors. So far, however, this has not translated into an improvement in outcome. This is different from what has been observed for the combination of radiation and hormonal therapy.

Unfortunately, about 20 to 30 percent of patients will demonstrate a rising PSA in the years following surgery. A majority of these patients will not have cancer at the margins of their prostate or cancer in their lymph nodes. This makes many doctors speculate that in some patients, the disease can spread microscopically to distant lymph nodes or to the bone marrow even though it seems to be confined within the prostate.

Who should consider prostate surgery? Radical prostatectomy makes sense for generally healthy and relatively young men, usually age seventy and younger, with early-stage cancer. It is generally accepted that the risks of the procedure are not warranted if life expectancy is less than ten years.

Who should avoid prostate surgery? For patients with advanced cancers that have spread beyond the prostate, surgery is usually not performed regardless of age or cardiac risk status because it is thought that the operation would have little curative value. Patients who have conditions that make surgery a risk because of specific health problems are also not candidates for surgery. These include men with cardiac, vascular, or pulmonary disease, for whom the risk of anesthesia is such that they could have strokes or heart attacks either during or just after the procedure. Patients that might have any of these conditions are often referred to a specific specialist such as a cardiologist to "clear" them for surgery. In addition, because of the relatively long recovery time, traditional surgery may not be the best alternative for men whose jobs require physical activity. (Men who cannot remain inactive during the recovery period may want to consider laparoscopic prostatectomy, described below.)

Advantages of prostate surgery. Surgery allows for the immediate removal of the cancer. This often is important psychologically. The procedure has a long track record of success and is often called the gold standard of primary treatments. Although a true head-to-head comparison with radiation therapy has not been performed, many believe that surgery holds the best chance for long-term cure. Also, the full extent of the disease within the gland can be assessed by the pathologist after surgery. This not only has prognostic significance, but also sometimes diagnostic implications; if the disease is of a higher stage or grade, sometimes further therapy might be considered.

Disadvantages of prostate surgery. Prostate surgery, like any surgery, has certain serious risks. They include the following:

• *Impotence.* The nerves that stimulate erections run adjacent to the prostate on their way to the penis. Normally, these nerves are cut during surgery removing the prostate, resulting in impotence. In certain circumstances, doctors can perform nerve-sparing procedures, in which the nerves going to the penis on the side of the prostate are identified and spared. Not every male is a good candidate for nerve-sparing surgery; it depends on the extent and location of the disease. The procedure is more successful in younger men. Older men, especially if they are already experiencing some degree of impotence, may not have very good results from nerve sparing.

I am often asked why urologists don't use nerve-sparing procedures on all patients. The reason is that for patients with more extensive cancer within their prostate glands, the operation might actually be "cancer sparing," by leaving some cancer behind after the surgery.

Men who develop impotence may be treated after surgery with vacuum pumps, instillation of drugs into the penis, and prosthetics. If the nerves are cut, medications such as Viagra usually don't work. On the other hand, drugs like Viagra may be very useful in men with nerve-sparing prostate surgery.

You need to discuss the risks with your doctor prior to surgery, making clear the definitions of impotence (anything less than an erection capable of achieving penetration). It is difficult for your doctor to give an overall success rate, because patients vary so much. Still, he or she may be able to give you an idea of your chances of maintaining potency. Just remember that your surgeon often will not be able to assess whether or not you can undergo nerve-sparing surgery until the time of the operation.

• *Incontinence.* Immediately after removal of the catheter, most men will experience urinary incontinence and require some form of protection, such as an adult incontinence pad. Within three weeks, most men have achieved reasonably good control and require minimum protection. However, some 1 to 4 percent of men have permanent problems with urinary control and require some form of protection (diaper or pads). Up to 8 percent of men have mild incontinence, defined as leaking a few drops of urine. When discussing the risk of incontinence with your doctor, ask about the specific definition of the condition. Also ask your doctor about his or her incontinence rate. Unfortunately, there may be no way of verifying this information, so you need to trust your surgeon.

• *Long convalescence period.* Vigorous physical activity must be restricted for about six weeks. You should not lift anything thirty pounds or heavier for four to six months, so forget yard work or lifting older grandchildren. An intensive strain can re-open the incision.

• *Blood loss.* Most men lose more than one unit of blood during a radical prostatectomy; on some occasions, the blood loss can be more than three or four units. If you plan to have surgery, you might consider an autologous transfusion, storing your own blood in the weeks beforehand so that you can receive it if needed in surgery. (Although this process may delay surgery by several weeks, the delay is not likely to be critical. Again, ask your surgeon about this.)

Tell your surgeon about any other prior surgeries you have had. It is important for him to know if you have had any problems with excessive bleeding during these past surgeries, or even during dental work. Patients on blood thinners might not be good candidates for surgery unless their medication can be stopped for a time.

• *Surgical and anesthetic complications.* Pain, infection, anesthetic problems, pneumonia, blood clots, and heart problems can occur with any major operation. Men who undergo prostatectomy also have a very slight risk of injury to the rectum and scarring of the new connection between the bladder and urethra.

Types of Prostate Surgery

There are several different types of prostatectomies:

Radical retropubic prostatectomy (RRP) is one of the most common types of surgery for prostate cancer. It involves cutting into the lower abdomen and then completely excising (or removing) the prostate.

Radical perineal prostatectomy (RPP): During this procedure, the prostate is removed through an incision in the perineum (the area of tissue between the scrotum and the anus). With RPP, major abdominal surgery and the risk of hernia can be avoided, but there is still a painful incision.

Laparoscopic prostatectomy: This procedure uses a smaller incision and fiber-optic scopes to perform the surgery. It has a shorter recovery time than traditional surgery, and, because of the smaller incision, patients are allowed to lift much sooner. Because this is a relatively new technique, studies are ongoing to compare the success rate of laparoscopic and traditional surgery. You should be sure your surgeon is very well versed in the technique before considering this option. (See the next chapter for more information.)

Radiation

This form of therapy involves exposing cancer cells to high doses of radiation that kill the cells and shrink the tumor. In some cases of cancer, doctors recommend radiation after surgery, to ensure that all malignant cells have been destroyed. Other times radiation is used instead of surgery.

Two general types of radiation therapy are used for prostate cancer: external-beam radiation and brachytherapy (seed implants).

External-beam radiation is administered to a small area of the abdomen and used to reach the prostate and sometimes the surrounding lymph nodes. This procedure takes about five to ten minutes, and it is repeated four or five days a week for seven or eight weeks. The radiation is aimed at the prostate from many different angles in an attempt to reduce the radiation exposure to the surrounding tissues. For patients with more advanced disease and some chance of lymph node involvement (according to the Partin tables in Appendix B), the radiologist might suggest pelvic radiation. This results in a bigger field than treatment of the prostate only.

External-beam radiation therapy is often delivered using 3-D techniques, which help deliver the radiation precisely to the desired field. Another recent development involves the use of intensity-modulated radiation therapy (IMRT), which allows doctors to better administer higher doses of radiation while sparing normal tissues.

Yet another increasingly popular method of treatment involves combined seed therapy (described below) and external-beam therapy. The idea is that external-beam therapy is given for five to six weeks instead of seven to eight, thereby decreasing the chance for rectal or bladder toxicity. The seed therapy seems to give the necessary boost to the prostate, resulting in a good anticancer therapy.

External-beam therapy is also given as a form of salvage therapy after radical prostatectomy. It may be recommended in two different situations. First, it may be advised if there is evidence that traces of cancer were left behind after surgery. This is often described as a positive margin, meaning the scalpel may have cut through the cancer, leaving some of it behind.

The other situation may occur many months after the surgery. If a man's PSA level rises again after surgery, and there is no other evidence of metastatic disease, radiation therapy to the pelvis may be recommended, even though it is impossible to know if the cancerous cells exist in the pelvis or a more distant site. In this case, if the PSA becomes undetectable and stays that way, the salvage radiation was successful; if the PSA continues to rise, it can be assumed that cancerous cells had escaped to another part of the body. Obviously, sometimes PSA levels decrease but only transiently, suggesting that there is cancer both in the pelvis and also at distant sites.

Interstital brachytherapy radiation involves implanting small radioactive seeds directly into the prostate. This procedure is done through the perineum and is guided by ultrasound. The operation can last from one to two hours, and requires anesthesia. It is followed by a hospital stay of several hours or overnight. Most implants are left in place (iodine, palladium, gold); others are temporary (iridium). Implants allow higher doses of radiation to reach the cancer cells within the prostate while sparing the surrounding tissues. The radiation is measured in concentric circles, and the depth of penetration of the radiation is measured in millimeters.

Adjuvant or neoadjuvant hormonal therapy is often begun prior to radiation therapy. As discussed on page 73, hormonal therapy for prostate cancer generally involves either inhibiting

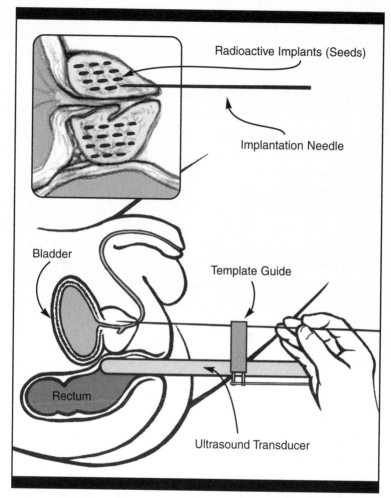

Figure 5.1 During brachytherapy, a radiation oncologist inserts radioactive seeds into the prostate using an ultrasound transducer to guide the needle for accurate placement.

the production of testosterone or blocking its effects. When hormonal therapy is recommended with radiation therapy, the therapy generally inhibits testosterone production. It is given in conjunction with radiation therapy in one of two ways. The first way it's given is prior to seed therapy, in order to shrink the prostate to allow more effective seed placement. This is because prostate glands of a certain size (about sixty grams) are too large to effectively seed without hormone therapy.

In cases of more advanced prostate cancer, hormonal therapy may be started about two months prior to external-beam therapy and continue for at least two months or more after its completion. This is done for patients who are not good candidates for brachytherapy because of the extent of their disease. This is a form of neoadjuvant or adjuvant (helper) therapy to improve the effects of external-beam radiation therapy so it is more effective. Studies have shown that hormonal therapy, when given as an adjuvant with external beam radiation therapy, improves the radiation therapy's overall effectiveness.

Who should consider radiation therapy? There are a number of good reasons to consider radiation therapy. For patients with more advanced prostate cancer (those with a Gleason pattern of 4 + 3 or higher, PSA values of more than 10, multiple core biopsies positive for cancer, or stage T3 disease), external-beam radiation therapy may be superior to radical prostatectomy, especially when combined with hormonal therapy. For patients with prostate cancer that is less aggressive (normal digital rectal exam, PSA values of less than 10, a Gleason pattern of 3 + 3 or 3 + 4, and few cores positive for cancer), seed therapy might be a preferred form of radiation therapy. Radiation therapy is also recommended for older patients or those with conditions that might result in problems during surgery. The latter includes forms of heart or lung disease, risk of stroke, and bleeding disorders.

Who should avoid radiation therapy? Radiation should probably be avoided by men who have a history of colon cancer or other bowel disorders because the treatment can exacerbate bowel problems.

Advantages of radiation therapy. External-beam radiation therapy may be more effective than surgery when the cancer has spread beyond the prostate, especially if combined with hormone therapy. It also allows men to avoid the side effects inevitable with surgery.

Some men choose surgery over radiation so that radiation can be used as salvage therapy if the cancer returns after surgery. It is not clear to me how much this should sway an individual's choice, because salvage therapy, at least for a rising PSA, is often not successful. It is my belief that after a well-performed prostatectomy, a patient with a rising PSA is unlikely to have local cancer only.

The situation can be explained this way: Roughly one-third of men will demonstrate PSA progression after radical prostatectomy. Of those men, optimistically speaking, one-third (likely even less than that) will have a five-year period of undetectable PSA values after salvage radiation therapy. This means that only about 10 percent of men will benefit altogether from salvage radiation therapy.

Recently a retrospective study published in the *Journal of the American Medical Association* suggested that patients with lower Gleason scores and longer PSA doubling times were more likely to have good responses to salvage radiation therapy for rising PSA values after prostatectomy.

Disadvantages of radiation therapy. External-beam radiation treatments in the short run can cause diarrhea, rectal pain, urinary urgency, and incontinence. During the last two or three weeks of treatment, symptoms are quite common and infrequently become so severe that the treatments must be temporarily halted. These symptoms usually disappear a few weeks after the final treatment, but a small percentage of men experience chronic rectal pain and urinary problems. Radiation can also eventually result in impotence due to scarring of nearby blood vessels. About one out of every two men who receive external-beam radiation also experience impotence, but often years after therapy. Many of these cases respond to treatment with Viagra.

Your doctor cannot predict how sensitive your rectum may be to radiation exposure. Very few men—about 1 percent—will have painful defecation. Radiation "scatter" can also damage the bladder. In most cases, the symptoms disappear, but for some men the damage is lifelong. The radiation may leave the bladder unable to hold sufficient urine, so that it is necessary for men to have to urinate very frequently, both day and night. Another concern for patients undergoing radiation therapy is the risk of cancers caused by the radiation. This is a rare event, but it can happen.

It is essential that you work with a radiation oncologist with expertise in handling prostate cancer. Improperly placed seeds can cause incomplete destruction of the cancer. There can also be damage to the lining of the rectum, causing urine to pass through the bowel and feces to pass through the urinary tract. These side effects appear less likely to occur, however, when interstitial radiation is correctly performed by a highly qualified physician.

FOLLOW-UP TREATMENT

No matter which primary treatment you and your doctor choose, you will be monitored closely during the months after the procedure. Every visit should include a digital rectal exam of the prostate or, in the case of men who have had the prostate surgically removed, an exam of the area where the prostate used to be. The doctor will be feeling for evidence of recurrence or return of the tumor. If suspicious areas occur, ultrasound and biopsies may be indicated.

In addition, expect to have ongoing PSA blood tests. After the prostate gland is removed, PSA levels should drop to undetectable (less than 0.1). If PSA levels are detected after radical prostatectomy (especially if the level rises to above 0.5), then we assume that there are prostate cancer cells somewhere in the body. It is somewhat frustrating, however, because given current radiographic techniques we cannot determine whether the cancer is in the prostate bed, the lymph nodes, or outside the pelvis. If the cancer is in the pelvis only, it might respond to salvage radiation therapy.

Recurrent cancer may require other treatments.

Hormonal Treatment

Hormone therapy is a misnomer; it should be called *hormone-removal therapy*, because it usually blocks or removes the effects of testosterone, which is necessary for most prostate cancers to grow. Although hormone therapy can be used in conjunction with primary therapies, it is also used as salvage treatment if surgery or radiation has failed. As a general rule, this type of therapy involves periodic injections, either monthly or every three to four months, or the use of oral therapy in the form of pills.

For decades, estrogen-based drugs were used in hormone therapy to reduce testosterone levels. But these estrogenic drugs had a wide range of side effects, including breast enlargement, hair loss, weight gain, hot flashes, impotence, loss of sexual desire, heart irregularities, blood clots, and stroke. To avoid some of these unwanted side effects, men opted for the surgical removal of their testicles (orchiectomy), which effectively eliminated the major source of testosterone production and reduced the chance of blood clots and stroke.

Today, these approaches have been replaced by the use of a new breed of hormonal therapies that use antiandrogenic drugs. There are two main classes of antiandrogenic drugs: luteinizing hormone-releasing hormone analogs (LHRH analogs), which fool the pituitary gland into halting testosterone production in the testes and are given by injection; and antiandrogens, which block testosterone's ability to bind to testosterone receptors and are given as pills. In the past, it was thought that when these therapies were combined it would result in a longer duration of response. However, many physicians do not think this is the case, and this so-called complete androgen blockade (CAB) approach is not used very much today.

The LHRH analogs lower testosterone to the same levels achieved by orchiectomy, and they are not associated with thrombosis (blood clots) as is the case with estrogen therapy. The side effects of any testosterone-lowering therapy are the same, however, regardless of how achieved. In the short run (about two or three weeks into treatment), patients might experience hot flashes and fatigue. Almost all patients will also experience loss of libido and impotence. This treatment is also associated with weight gain of about five or six pounds. In the long run, testosterone-lowering therapy is associated with bone loss (osteoporosis) and muscle wasting. Bone loss can be altered with the use of bisphosphonates such as Fosamax, which is an oral agent, or Zometa (zoledronic acid) or Aredia (pamidronate), which are intravenous medications.

Another problem: LHRH analogs are associated with an initial surge in testosterone. If a patient has metastatic bone disease, this surge can be associated with increased pain or even spinal cord compression, because the surge in testosterone causes the cancer to grow. To try to prevent this problem, it is recommended that physicians administer an antiandrogen in combination with LHRH analogs for the first few weeks of therapy. A newer alternative, however, is the use of an LHRH antagonist called Plenaxis. This therapy, given every two weeks and then monthly, results in an immediate decrease in testosterone levels without any initial spike in testosterone.

The other form of hormonal therapy, antiandrogens, has fewer side effects but is generally not as effective as testosterone-lowering therapies. These therapies, when used without testosterone-lowering therapy, do not usually have a major effect on libido or bone loss. They are associated with breast enlargement and breast swelling. This can be so severe that it is sometimes recommended that men undergo a short course of prophylactic radiation therapy to the breast to avoid the problem.

As discussed previously, hormone therapy is sometimes used before radiation or surgery to initially shrink the tumors. Smaller tumors allow the radiation to be more tightly focused, with fewer side effects. Currently hormonal therapy is used most frequently for men with rising PSA values but no signs of metastasis. It is also given to men who do have metastatic disease as well as rising PSA levels. It is simply not known if giving "early" hormonal therapy is preferable to waiting for signs of metastasis. You should discuss this decision with your physician and ask him which protocol he prefers and why.

While very successful in most men, the benefits of hormone therapy last only a few years. Between 80 and 90 percent of men receiving hormone treatment (including surgical removal of the testes) will have an initial reduction in PSA levels, and in tumor size, if a tumor is present. However, within two to three years the cancer will become refractory, meaning that it begins to grow again. While researchers do not fully understand the process, we do know that tumors that are refractory to hormonal therapy become increasingly made up of androgen-insensitive cells that have replaced the original androgen-sensitive ones.

Who should consider hormone therapy? This approach is often recommended when the cancer has spread beyond the prostate, or if a man experiences a recurrence of cancer after a first round of radiation or surgery. It is also used for men with symptomatic metastatic disease.

Who should avoid hormone therapy? Hormone therapy is not recommended for localized cancer that is likely to be cured with surgery or radiation therapy alone.

It is not known why patients become refractory to hormonal therapy. There have been many explanations for this problem, including mutations in the androgen receptor or overexpression of the receptor. It is obvious that there are likely to be many causes, even in the same patient. Understanding the mechanism for why men become refractory offers the promise of better treatment, so this is an important area of research.

How Hormonal Treatments Work

While all hormonal treatments alter the balance of hormones in the body, different drugs are used to generate different effects.

Antiandrogens

- Drugs: Bicalutamide (Casodex), flutamide (Eulexin), nilutamide (Nilandron).

- What they do: They prevent dihydrotestosterone from binding to its receptor.

Estrogens

- Drugs: Diethylstilbesterol (DES).
- What it does: It inhibits the release of luteinizing hormone–releasing hormone from the hypothalamus and decreases testosterone levels.

Luteinizing Hormone–Releasing Hormone Analogs

- Drugs: Leuprolide (Lupron Depot), goserelin acetate (Zoladex), nafarelin (Synarel).
- What they do: They simulate excessive LHRH production, causing the hypothalamus to stop its signal for the production of LH from the pituitary thereby lowering testosterone production from the testes.

LHRH Antagonists

- Drugs: Plenaxis.
- What it does: This agent has just been approved to treat bone metastases. This is because the testosterone surge from LHRH analogs can have devastating effects.

5-Alpha Reductase Inhibitors

- Drugs: Finasteride (Proscar) or dutasteride (Avodart).
- What they do: These 5-alpha reductase inhibitors decrease the conversion of testosterone to DHT.

Adrenal Hormone-Synthesis Inhibitors

- Drugs: Ketoconazole, aminoglutethimide.

- What they do: They inhibit adrenal synthesis of testosterone and other steroids. These are given after LHRH analogs or orchiectomy, if antiandrogens stop working.

Chemotherapy

Chemotherapy is almost never used as the initial treatment of prostate cancer, even if advanced. It is mostly used for disease that progresses despite one or more hormonal therapies.

Chemotherapy involves the use of medicines to stop the growth of cancers. Chemotherapy drugs work by killing cells that tend to grow quickly. While cancer cells fit this description, so do cells in the bone marrow, the gastrointestinal tract, and hair follicles, which explains why many people who receive chemotherapy experience weakness, nausea, and hair loss.

Unfortunately, chemotherapy rarely cures prostate cancer; instead, it slows the rate of growth.

Until recently, chemotherapy was not prescribed for prostate cancer patients, but it has been more widely used in the last few years. For decades, chemotherapy brought with it all its negative side effects, without increasing survival rates. However, recent studies of one agent, mitoxantrone have found that the drug helps palliate pain associated with prostate cancer after it has spread to the bones, without causing side effects so severe that it adversely affects quality of life. This drug does not improve the survival rate of men with advanced metastatic prostate cancer, but it does ameliorate, at least for a while, many of their symptoms.

Other drugs under investigation hold promise. For example, tests using taxane-based drugs (Taxol and Taxotere) show that these agents, especially Taxotere, extend life in men with late-stage disease. Therefore, taxane-based regimens are now most commonly used for hormone-refractory disease.

Other studies under way involve the use of chemotherapy

drugs in conjunction with other therapies. One study in progress compares two groups of men who have had radical prostatectomy, but have adverse risk factors for recurrence. One group of men will receive two years of hormone therapy following the surgery; another will receive six months of chemotherapy and then two years of hormone therapy following the surgery. If the research shows that the chemotherapy improves the outcomes in late-stage disease, then researchers will look at the impact the drugs can have at earlier stages of disease. Finally, newer agents, many of which are described in chapter 6, are being used in combination with taxane-based chemotherapy.

Who should consider chemotherapy? Chemotherapy drugs may make patients with late-stage disease feel better, and they may change survival rates. These drugs are used most frequently after hormonal therapies are exhausted.

Who should avoid chemotherapy? Men who cannot tolerate the side effects of the treatment should avoid chemotherapy. Unless as part of an experiment, men who do not have symptoms from prostate cancer should avoid chemotherapy until they become symptomatic.

Advantages of chemotherapy. This treatment can provide pain relief in men whose cancer has spread to the bone. Some drugs under investigation may help extend the lives of men with advanced prostate cancer.

Disadvantages of chemotherapy. Common complications of chemotherapy include anemia, weakness, nausea, vomiting, diarrhea, mouth sores, hair loss, and low white blood cell counts. Patients who are offered chemotherapy need to discuss the side effects of specific agents with their doctors. Some agents, such as mitoxantrone, are relatively benign. Others have many more side effects. Patients need to know that chemotherapy is not one "thing." It is important to explore the side effects of any regimen prior to beginning therapy.

*   *   *

Some men experience a recurrence of prostate cancer after the traditional follow-up therapies have been exhausted. For these men, many new therapies are available. Chapter 6 will help you weigh the pros and cons of different treatment options in your particular case. In addition, it will discuss experimental therapies for prostate cancer that appear to hold promise for men whose cancer returns after primary and salvage therapy.

What Most Doctors Won't Tell You: Experimental Treatments Your Doctor May Not Know About

For most men, prostate cancer will be a single chapter—and not the final chapter—in their lives. Although the experience may be terrifying and life altering, most men will respond well to conventional treatment and eventually declare themselves prostate-cancer-free survivors. These men will never need to turn to experimental or investigational treatments for prostate cancer.

Some men, however, will find that their cancer recurs, sometimes again and again, and each time a man must work with his doctor to further explore the therapeutic options. About one-third of men who receive primary therapy for their prostate cancer will at some point experience another rise in their PSA, indicating a return of the cancer. For most of these men, no immediate therapy is necessary, and some, based on PSA doubling time, might never need therapy. Others will eventually require some form of therapy, usually hormonal.

However, as discussed above, hormone therapies are almost always finite in their duration of effectiveness. When they are no longer working, there are a number of conventional therapies available, including secondary forms of hormone therapy, chemotherapy, or salvage radiation therapy in men who have not tried radiation previously.

At many times during the progression of the disease, a patient may be eligible for a specific clinical trial. Men usually enroll in a clinical trial to receive drugs that are in the experimental stages of development. (For more information on deciding whether or not to participate in a clinical trial, see chapter 7.)

Experimental treatments exist in a gray area, using therapies that have not yet been proven successful for a specific stage of prostate cancer. These treatments will shape the future treatment of prostate cancer; they are the ultimate source of optimism for many patients who have started to lose hope for remission. On the other hand, too often people see experimental treatments as a final lifeline, a last chance for life; most treatments can't live up to those high expectations.

Literally dozens of new agents and combinations of agents for the treatment of prostate cancer are in development; a few of these agents will work, but most of them will be ineffective or have so many dangerous side effects that they will create more problems than they solve. Still, even methods that fail help broaden our understanding of prostate cancer; we learn as much from our failures as we do from our successes.

I specialize in the treatment of prostate cancer, yet even I find it difficult to keep up with every trial going on for prostate cancer in this country. For the general oncologist who treats other forms of cancer as well, it is all but impossible to know about every trial and form of treatment under investigation for prostate cancer. For this reason, some highly qualified urologists and oncologists may not be informed about some of the innovative trials currently in progress.

In my experience, most doctors do not feel defensive toward patients who bring in information they have collected from books or the Internet. It is my opinion that it is your disease and your body, and you have a right to learn as much as you choose to about possible treatments.

This chapter will highlight some of the more promising treatments for prostate cancer currently in development. The following chapter will help you decide if a clinical trial is right for you. Given the vast amount of ongoing research on prostate cancer, this section will be current only at the time of publication.

A TALE OF CAUTION: THE PC-SPES EXPERIENCE

I have learned a lot from my experience with the herbal formula known as PC-SPES. (The *PC* stands for "prostate cancer"; *spes* is the Latin word for "hope.") The formula was popularized by a chemist named Sophie Chen, Ph.D., who claimed the treatment integrated modern Western science and ancient Chinese herbal wisdom. In the 1990s, PC-SPES was considered an alternative medicine breakthrough; today, it is no longer on the market.

For me, the story began in 1996 when a former patient came from Chicago to see me. This man had been diagnosed with advanced metastatic prostate cancer when he'd been my patient several years before; I prescribed hormone treatment (Lupron injections), and he was doing well five or six years later. In 1996, he told me he had been taking PC-SPES, which he bought from a place in California for about four hundred dollars a month. I would have dismissed his claims as a scam, but then he showed me his records. His PSA level had been

150 when he started on the PC-SPES, and two months later it was 25. He had been taking two or three Percocet painkillers every day, and now he was off them altogether. I took notice.

I asked him to bring me his pills, as well as everything else he was taking. I copied the label, but I wasn't familiar with the herbs and other ingredients, except for saw palmetto, which I knew could not by itself have caused such a dramatic reversal in symptoms. The herbs included chrysanthemum (or mum), the stem of reishi, the root of baikal skullcap, licorice, *Ganoderma lucidum,* Panax ginseng, San Qi ginseng, the leaf of *Rabdosia rubescens,* saw palmetto, and the leaf of Dyers wood. These are not compounds that we learned about in medical school pharmacology classes.

I began asking all my patients to bring me the bottles of every supplement they were taking. Several other patients were taking the same PC-SPES, and they also demonstrated a decrease in their PSA levels. Many men with advanced cancer experienced less pain and needed lower doses of narcotics. After more than two decades of clinical experience, I believe I can usually tell whether a patient is getting better or worse, and these men were getting better.

I felt I was no longer in a position to dismiss this alternative medication. I discussed PC-SPES with other academic oncologists who specialize full-time in the treatment of late-stage prostate cancer, and their experiences were similar. We pooled our knowledge—or ignorance, in this case—and we quickly realized that there was something to PC-SPES.

Medicine is a two-way street: Patients learn from their doctors, and doctors learn from their patients. If my patients want to try PC-SPES or some other alternative treatment, I can't just dismiss their desires out of hand. However, I can't promise them that the alternative will work or that they will not experience side effects. Because most alternative medicines have not gone through the battery of tests for safety and efficacy required of traditional medicines, my colleagues and I were unaware of all the side effects or potential drug interactions possible with PC-SPES. After explaining these caveats to my patients, I always encourage them to tell me about all of the alternative treatments they are using so that I can monitor their medical condition.

I have had the occasional patient who feels the need to choose between conventional and alternative medicine, although I do not believe most patients must select one or the other. One man in my care moved to El Salvador to receive intravenous infusions of an herbal treatment. Within one month his PSA level shot up from 1 to 50. He abandoned the alternative treatment and returned to my practice. I understand his need to seek out new medical therapies and alternatives, but I don't believe you should abandon conventional medicine. Every patient deserves the best treatments available to him, without becoming dogmatic about following one approach or another.

Some doctors give patients the implicit message that if they try alternative treatments, the physician will no longer treat them. I would only feel that way if traditional medicine had a definitive cure to offer. When a man experiences recurrent prostate cancer after hormone therapy, we have quite a few treatments to try, but conventional medicine has its limits and does not typically offer anything like a "cure." In the absence of curative therapy, I think alternative therapies are unlikely to cause harm if a patient is monitored carefully for effectiveness and side effects during a two-month trial period. Men should, however, be cautious. Sadly, there are unethical people who prey on desperate cancer patients, who are willing to pay high prices and try almost anything to save their lives.

When it comes to PC-SPES, the treatment was not a hoax,

but it did not live up to its initial promise. It didn't cure people, but it gave people with late-stage, hormonal-refractory disease some months of life they might not have had. They did, however, experience side effects, including breast enlargement and tenderness. More important, PC-SPES increased a man's risk of stroke and deep-vein thrombosis, potentially life-threatening side effects that could be countered with blood-thinning medications.

There wasn't anything in the medical literature about PC-SPES until the mid-1990s. We found that almost one in two men who were hormone refractory (their PSA levels were rising even though they had low testosterone levels) responded to the PC-SPES. This was surprising, since PC-SPES was not simply working by lowering testosterone, although it had that effect as well in men who had not been on Lupron. Therefore, the benefit of PC-SPES treatment did not result solely from its ability to lower hormone levels.

The effectiveness of PC-SPES in some patients who were hormone refractory was very intriguing. My colleagues here in Boston and San Francisco designed a trial comparing men on DES (a synthetic estrogen) to men on PC-SPES. Both groups were also treated with blood thinner to counter the blood-clotting side effects of both agents. When men progressed by PSA or clinical criteria, we switched their therapy to the other in a crossover design to find out if the men might respond to the other agent. In the first part of the trial, PC-SPES proved to be better than DES. About half the men responded to the PC-SPES and only one-quarter to the DES.

During the study, we heard reports that there were variations among different batches of PC-SPES. Therefore, we analyzed lots of PC-SPES using high-performance liquid chromatography, a technique that separates by molecular weight every compound in the mixture. In two of the four batches tested, the "natural" PC-SPES contained a small amount of diethylstilbestrol and possibly the blood thinner warfarin, both prescription drugs. Clearly, there were problems with both contamination and quality control. The authorities at both Harvard and the University of California at San Francisco who oversee clinical trials stopped the study. The California Attorney General banned the sale of the product because it was a drug, not an herb.

This PC-SPES experience illustrates one of the major problems with testing herbal remedies. Batch-to-batch variations make quality control very difficult. Medicinal plants play a critical role in healing; Taxol and digitalis are two of many important drugs first derived from plants. In most cases, medicinal plants are studied, and the active components isolated and adapted into synthetic drugs so that the active components can be administered accurately.

Although PC-SPES was an over-the-counter herbal treatment, it proved to be both effective—and somewhat dangerous. In men who had not tried conventional hormone therapy, it could have interfered with their ability to respond at a later time because their tumors might have become unresponsive to hormone treatment. Alternative medicines may play a role in the treatment of prostate disease (as described later in this book), but treatments such as PC-SPES that promise miracle cures should be approached with skeptical curiosity.

PROMISING TREATMENTS IN DEVELOPMENT

The following is a summary of some of the leading treatments for prostate cancer that remain in the experimental stages.

Local Experimental Therapies

Hyperthermia

Hyperthermia involves the use of heat to kill cancer cells. It is often performed to enhance the effectiveness of traditional radiation therapy. One of the advantages of this dual approach is that smaller-than-normal amounts of radiation can be used to shrink tumors.

Various techniques are used in hyperthermia. One involves the insertion of plastic or fiber-optic cylinders into the prostate; bursts of microwave or ultrasound energy are then delivered through the cylinders directly into the tumors. Another technique uses magnetic rods or sapphire probes to deliver laser-generated heat to tumors. The technique is currently being tested in a few clinical trials.

Who might benefit? Hyperthermia is only useful for patients who need local therapy. If you're interested in hyperthermia, seek treatment from a radiation oncologist who has extensive experience in this form of treatment. At present, this treatment must be performed as part of a clinical trial. This approach is being tested most in men with aggressive cancers, as measured by high Gleason scores.

Cryosurgery

Cryosurgery (also known as cryoablation or cryotherapy) treats localized prostate cancer (cancer that has not spread beyond the prostate) by freezing prostate cells to destroy them. During the procedure, a five- or eight-pronged probe filled with nitrogen is inserted through a small incision in the perineum and placed into the cancerous area in the prostate. The probe, which is guided by a transrectal ultrasound, then releases nitrogen or argon gas, dropping the temperature in the prostate to as low as –195 degrees Celsius. At the same time, a catheter is used to warm the urethra to prevent damage. The freezing continues for about an hour as an "ice ball" forms around the prostate.

Research involving cryotherapy procedures in the early 1990s did not yield impressive results. Two years after treatment, 20 percent of the men treated with the five-probe method had positive biopsies, and 70 percent had detectable PSA levels. The best of the studies showed that 30 percent of men had elevated PSA levels four years after treatment.

There are no long-term studies comparing the effectiveness of cryotherapy (as either a first- or second-line therapy) to traditional surgery or radiation therapy. The procedure has been refined since its introduction, however, specifically by increasing the number of probes and changing from argon gas to liquid nitrogen as the coolant. In most cases, cryosurgery is used as a secondary therapy following radiation treatment.

I have seen wide differences in outcomes following cryosurgery. Undoubtedly, some of the differences are based on the doctor's experience. The procedure has several benefits, including low morbidity with the technique, minimal blood loss, and a short hospital stay.

On the other hand, some of the worst cases of incontinence I have ever seen have involved men who had cryosurgery. A large U.S. study of cryotherapy patients found that up to 27 percent experienced incontinence following the procedure. In addition, the same study found other side effects, including impotence (40 to 80 percent of men) and temporary penile numbness and swelling (up to 10 percent). Also, damage to the urethra can in rare cases cause the passing of urine through the bowel.

Who might benefit? Men with local prostate disease who have had radiation are not candidates for traditional surgery as salvage therapy. Some of these men can try cryosurgery with the hope that this will render them free of disease. However, interview your doctors extensively prior to the procedure and choose a physician with extensive experience using this technique. Doctors who perform cryosurgery should have in-depth and long-term experience with the procedure. Talk to support groups and other survivors to get the names of doctors who are recommended. You do not need to participate in a clinical trial to receive cryosurgery.

Laparoscopic Prostatectomy

Laparoscopic surgery is performed with the aid of a device that can look into the body and perform surgery while only a small incision is made in the skin. Laparoscopic procedures tend to involve less blood loss and a decreased need for painkillers than do traditional surgical methods. The procedure has gained popularity for removing the gallbladder and for other routine procedures in the abdominal cavity.

In recent years, the approach has been used for the removal of the prostate. Data on the effectiveness of the procedure in the treatment of prostate cancer are not available yet. Some experts express concern that the surgeon may need a more precise visual image to eradicate the cancer with confidence.

Who might benefit? Laparoscopic prostatectomy may be worth considering by men with localized cancer who need to resume physical activity as soon as possible after surgery, perhaps due to the demands of a job. The convalescence may be easier for most men. Patients interested in the procedure should interview surgeons with extensive experience using the technique. Laparoscopic surgery is not considered experimental.

Systemic Therapies

Immunotherapy (Vaccine Therapy)

Immune-based therapies are directed at stimulating your own immune system to attack your prostate cancer. Several different immune-based strategies are now being tested. The goal of vaccine therapy is to get the body to recognize cancer cells as foreign, then attack and eliminate them. The problem is that our own immune system usually does not see cancer cells as foreign. Vaccine therapy attempts to train the immune system to recognize cancer cells (for instance, targeting cells that express PSA).

There is evidence that in advanced prostate cancer (as well as other cancers), a patient's immune system grows weaker at the time it is needed most. To jump-start the immune system, scientists have experimented with injecting granulocyte macrophage colony-stimulating factor (GM-CSF) directly into the tumor cells. This growth factor triggers a series of reactions that strengthen the immune system: It increases the number of dendritic cells, which in turn stimulate specific T cells, a type of lymphocyte that targets prostate and other cancer tumor cells.

There are currently several different experimental vaccine strategies undergoing evaluation. As will be discussed in the next chapter, it is important to read thoroughly and to understand the informed consent document you will sign before entering a clinical trial using a vaccine. All vaccine therapies are currently experimental, so you will need to enroll in a clinical trial.

One vaccine study was done on men who underwent radical prostatectomy or radiation therapy but experienced a rise in their PSA levels shortly thereafter. In an early trial of a "PSA" vaccine—one directed at stimulating the immune system to destroy cell expressions of PSA—sixteen of twenty-one men

Is It a Miracle?

In more than two decades of practice, I have had one patient go into unexplained spontaneous remission for prostate cancer. When he came to me, his PSA level was 52. We debated various treatment options, and he decided to have hormone therapy. Prior to starting treatment, we tested his PSA again; the level had dropped to 40. He had not received any hormones or medications. We continued to test his levels without treatment, and they dropped down to 5 and held steady.

I had another patient whose PSA levels also dropped, but additional studies detected a tumor in the pituitary gland of his brain that had blocked the production of testosterone. When the tumor was removed, the man's PSA levels rose again, and he needed hormone treatment.

We did a number of tests on the man with the spontaneous remission and could not find any tumors or other explanation for his change of health. He continues to survive, cancer-free.

who received the vaccine experienced slower PSA increases than could be expected without treatment. One patient had a seven-month reduction in his PSA. These responses are modest but do provide evidence that this approach may hold promise if it can be enhanced.

The PSA vaccine is now being tested in a larger group of patients. The concept is built around the smallpox vaccine, which is an inactivated version of the smallpox virus. When the body is exposed, it develops an immune response to the virus, but without the risk of developing the disease. For this vaccine, scientists removed some of the DNA of the smallpox virus and replaced it with the gene for PSA. The hope is that after vaccination, lymphocytes will target the PSA-producing cells.

I have administered this vaccine to a number of patients. Rare patients have had an excellent response with a decrease in PSA levels, and about 20 percent had PSA levels that remained flat; the rest did not respond.

Who might benefit? This treatment needs to be refined before it will be widely available. It will probably not be suitable for aggressive cancers, but it may be useful for men who experience rising PSA levels after surgery. At this point, it is available only in clinical trials.

Bone-directed medications

Prostate cancer typically spreads from the prostate to the lymph nodes or the bone marrow. The reason for the relatively specific spread of prostate cancer cells to these areas of the body is that there may be receptors on cells inside these areas that allow prostate cancer to enter the bone and divide. Bone-directed therapies attempt to make the bone an inhospitable environment for the cancer to grow in, potentially halting the progression of the cancer. By delaying the spread to the bone, patients with prostate cancer may be able to live longer and avoid or delay the excruciating pain of bone cancer.

There are several categories of bone-directed medications. They include:

- Atrasentan (an experimental drug that blocks a specific bone marrow receptor).[1]

[1] I am currently a paid consultant to Abbott Laboratories, the company developing Atrasentan. As such, I cannot perform clinical trials on this drug; I do not own stock in the company.

- Bisphosphonates (medications designed to strengthen the bones, to prevent osteoporosis and prevent bone pain in men with prostate cancer; these drugs also appear to make the bones less receptive to cancer cells). These drugs include Fosamax (oral), Aredia (intravenous), and Zometa (intravenous).

These medications typically are administered as a daily pill or an injection either monthly or every three months. The drugs appear to be well tolerated, and have shown to be useful for the treatment of other cancers as well. Bone-directed therapies may prove helpful in the men whose PSA levels rise following primary treatment to prevent or delay recurrence of cancer in the bone marrow.

There are clinical trials in progress to test these various therapies. If agents are already approved by the U.S. Food and Drug Administration—as are the bisphosphonates—they are often available to patients outside clinical studies. Agents that don't yet have FDA approval, such as Atrasentan, are available only in clinical trials.

Who might benefit? Bone-directed medications may prevent osteoporosis, a side effect of many hormonal therapies. They also may prevent the spread of cancer to the bone marrow.

Angiogenesis Inhibitors

These drugs restrict blood flow to tumors by interfering with the formation of new blood vessels, effectively starving them before they can grow and spread. Cancerous tumors rely on the formation of new vessels to satisfy their dramatic need for blood. By blocking the formation of new vessels, angiogenesis-inhibiting drugs may not at first destroy existing tumors, but they will prevent them from getting any larger and will over time result in cancer cell death.

The father of the field, Dr. Judah Folkman of Harvard Medical School, noted that adults grow vessels only during wound healing and with the formation of cancers. He isolated a number of compounds that inhibit vascular formation, without interfering with the preexisting vessels. The process of growing blood vessels is known as angiogenesis; drugs used to block this process are angiogenesis inhibitors.

Several antiangiogenesis drugs are being tested in the treatment of cancer, including angiostatin, endostatin, thalidomide, and others. Some of these are in clinical trials for prostate cancer. Some new agents are "natural" antiangiogenic agents isolated from part of a protein produced by the body. Others block receptors that promote angiogensis in blood vessel cells.

In the trials to date, the drugs that have been tested hold some promise, but they do not appear to be a magic bullet. This approach may work best for men with micrometastases (tiny tumors), but perhaps not when the cancer has become large enough to detect by X rays. They also may be more effective when used in combination with other agents. While the theory is intriguing, this strategy is still in its infancy.

Furthermore, unless the new agents kill all the tumor cells, these drugs may have to be used every day for the rest of a man's life to prevent the tumor from resuming its growth. One problem with this approach is that new blood vessels form in the heart as a natural way to bypass blocked vessels. There is concern that using these drugs on a prolonged basis could cause cardiovascular disease or problems with wound healing, but for now this does not seem to be a major obstacle to their use. Because these therapies are not yet approved, most are available only in clinical trials.

Who might benefit? Angiogenesis inhibitors are best suited for men whose cancer has spread beyond the prostate, but whose tumors are too small to be detected by X ray. (The new sites are identified only by rising PSA levels.)

Targeted Therapy

This approach involves the use of new drugs or new combinations of drugs to help treat advanced prostate cancer. Medical oncologists often look to existing chemotherapy agents and ask whether they can be altered or modified to improve their performance. Chemotherapy is particularly effective in cancers that attack rapidly dividing cells, but these drugs are sometimes less successful in the treatment of prostate cancer, possibly because prostate cancer cells tend to multiply fairly slowly.

Traditional chemotherapy agents inhibit cell function, but they aren't very good at identifying cancer cells. The next generation of chemotherapy drugs is designed to be like smart bombs, able to identify and act only when a cell expresses a certain protein. Some of the drugs in development will look for prostate-membrane-specific antigens, so that the only cells targeted by the drug will be prostate related. These drugs may be more effective, with fewer side effects.

Gleevec (imatinib) is an example of a new targeted drug that affects only cancer cells that express one of three growth factor receptors. One of these receptors is expressed in a form of chronic myelogenous leukemia (CML). Gleevec is very effective in this instance. Of course, growth factor receptors aren't the only targets to consider. Newer therapies target key proteins inside the cell that may lead to the proliferation or survival of cancer cells.

In the future, we hope to have the ability to take a blood

sample and determine precisely which proteins an individual's cancer is making so that we will know exactly how to treat it. The therapy will be individualized based on a number of factors, such as the pattern of growth factors expressed by a particular cancer. This approach may be a long way off, but the more we learn about particular cancers, the closer we are to being able to follow this customized approach.

Who might benefit? This therapy could be of use to any man with advanced prostate cancer. Clinical trials for certain agents, such as Gleevec, are currently taking place.

New Uses of Existing Drugs

While the previous section described new drugs in development, researchers also experiment with new combinations of existing drugs. For example, oncologists are using drugs known as taxanes for men with hormone-refractory and symptomatic prostate cancer, meaning that their cancer has returned after hormone therapy and they are experiencing bone pain, fatigue, weight loss, and other symptoms. When taken in combination with other drugs, especially an oral drug such as estramustine, taxanes have been proven to be effective. Studies performed with patients whose recurring cancer has spread to the bone have found that the use of taxanes with estramustine can lower PSA levels by 50 percent in 70 percent or more of patients.

The taxanes—Taxotere and Taxol—inhibit the ability of the cells to divide. They can be toxic to the nervous system; the most common symptom is neuropathy, often manifest as numbness in the feet. However, taxanes do play a role in the treatment of late-stage prostate cancer that no longer responds to other forms of treatment. Taxanes are not by themselves experimental; however, they are often used with other agents in new, experimental combinations.

Who might benefit? Men with recurrent cancer that has spread to the bone may benefit from the use of taxanes. Other drug combinations may prove helpful as well, depending on a man's particular cancer profile. Because these drugs have been approved for use with other cancers, they are available outside clinical trials. If a taxane is being used with an experimental agent or as part of an untested combination with other agents, you will be asked to sign an informed consent document. This means that this is experimental therapy.

Gene Therapy

The term *gene therapy* broadly refers to the process of changing the genetic makeup of the cancer cells or immune cells. Many of these therapies employ genetically engineered viruses, which look like regular viruses on the outside, but contain an altered genetic message on the inside. These viruses then attach to the prostate cells and destroy them, or identify them so that other drugs can locate them during search-and-destroy missions.

There is some hope for this strategy:

• According to the May 2001 issue of the journal *Human Gene Therapy*, researchers for the first time showed that immunotherapy delivered by gene therapy may help in the treatment of locally advanced prostate cancer. The study involved injecting gene-based immunotherapy using an ultrasound guidance system directly into the diseased prostate prior to surgery or after the failure of radiation therapy. Because it is injected into the prostate rather than throughout the system as a whole, there are few side effects. As part of the study, twenty-four patients with locally advanced prostate cancer (no metastases) were treated with gene-based immunotherapy using a gene that expressed interleukin-2 directly into the prostate.

This substance stimulates the immune system to attract "natural killer" cells called lymphocytes. More than half of the men in the study had reduced PSA levels. Although exciting, it is important to recognize the need for additional clinical trials, which are currently in progress. Also this strategy is only useful for local disease, and there is a much greater need for therapy directed at metastases.

• According to the April 2000 issue of *World Journal of Urology*, researchers at the University of Virginia laid a pre-clinical foundation for clinical trials targeting a bone protein that exists almost exclusively in tumors metastatic to bone, such as those found in prostate cancer patients. The strategy is for cells that take up the target to be destroyed by the drugs ganciclovir or acyclovir. This is because these cells now express a viral gene that forces the cancer cells to produce an enzyme called thymidine kinase, which is not normally found in healthy cells. Then the patient is given the drug acyclovir, which reacts with the thymidine kinase and converts the drug into a toxin that destroys the cancer cells. Research is in progress.

Dozens of clinical trials involving gene therapy are currently in progress, and many involve prostate cancer. While many of these treatments hold promise, most are probably years away from being widely available.

Who might benefit? This approach is currently most often tested in men with local cancers. Gene therapy and the other cutting-edge treatments under investigation are available only to men participating in clinical trials. A number of variables determine whether a man is qualified for a particular trial, including his stage of cancer and the treatments that have been attempted previously.

Should you participate in a clinical trial? The decision can be difficult, but the following chapter will help you weigh the advantages and disadvantages of joining a research project. It also will help you locate trials in progress so that you can find the right trial for your specific needs.

The Lazarus Syndrome

Early in my career, I had a patient with advanced cancer that had metastasized to the bones. His cancer was not detected until it was quite advanced and he had developed significant pain and a blood disorder. No one expected him to live long. Even though he was very ill when we started therapy, he responded dramatically to hormonal therapy and chemotherapy and almost experienced a Lazarus Syndrome. He lived seven years, most of which were completely pain-free. Seven years may not sound long to some people, but that was precious time he was able to spend with his family and loved ones.

I hope that in the coming years, we will experience more cases of the Lazarus Syndrome. A number of new treatments hold promise for turning prostate cancer into a chronic disease. Due to both early diagnosis and close follow-up after primary therapy, long-term survival appears to have already improved. New therapies, including those discussed in this chapter, are being developed, which may prolong the lives of prostate patients.

—○○○—

Chapter 7

New Hope or False Hope: Should You Participate in a Clinical Trial?

Some forms of prostate cancer can be defeated easily; others defy conventional treatments, returning time after time. For these persistent and pernicious cancers, traditional treatments are sometimes not enough. In such cases, the greatest hope often lies in clinical trials.

Clinical trials typically involve experimental procedures, medications, or combinations of medications. Some prostate cancer trials involve new treatments for advanced cancers, while others may involve new approaches to less aggressive cancers or even for prostate cancer prevention. Some men join trials because they have no other options; others want to further medical science and do not feel their lives depend on the outcome of the research. Still others are interested in a new treatment they may have read about that they hope will help them with some aspect of their care.

I believe that clinical trials are essential for the advancement of prostate cancer treatment. In my practice, I have enrolled many prostate cancer patients in a variety of clinical trials, many of which I have been involved in as an investigator. Trials are the primary mechanism a medical researcher has to test potential drugs and treatments to determine their safety and effectiveness.

When discussing clinical trials with my patients, I find that most patients have a preconceived bias. People tend to view clinical trials in dramatic terms, either imagining study participants being used as human guinea pigs to test dangerous, unapproved drugs, or envisioning test subjects as having the inside track on acquiring miracle medicines years before they are made available to the public.

In truth, clinical research is far more mundane than either extreme. While not free of all risk, clinical trials are typically quite safe. Checks and balances are built into the research process, often with oversight boards to monitor the trials and to protect the health of participants.

Clinical trials don't manufacture miracle cures, either. Cancer has been a difficult disease to treat, and progress is often only incremental. Some approaches will work with some men, but not others. Our goal as research scientists and clinical investigators is to come up with a variety of treatments that will work in men with a variety of cancer profiles.

Toward that end, clinical trials progress slowly from one stage to the next, usually starting with a theory and laboratory testing, then gradually moving into the realm of human research. In addition, it must be noted that many clinical trials simply refine existing treatment protocols, without exploring wholly new approaches to treatment.

On the other hand, a man with late-stage refractory (recurring) cancer may see a clinical trial as a last hope of prolonging life. Most of these men have undergone traditional treatments, but their cancer has returned. They may not have responded to hormonal treatments, or more typically they may find that the treatments are no longer working. For these men, clinical trials may offer hope of a new treatment that can help get their cancer back under control. For example, a man with hormone-refractory prostate cancer might participate in a study when he is no longer responding to treatment (as demonstrated by a rise in PSA, new bone lesions, or a new tumor).

As a doctor, it is difficult to help patients hold on to the promise of a cure without encouraging them to cling to false hope. While I share my patients' desire for a miraculous result, at this point I believe our greatest possibility of saving lives is by laboriously working on a variety of new treatments that may prolong the lives of some men, some of the time. Each new treatment may work for a few weeks or months before the cancer progresses, but if we have enough of these treatments available, the cancer can be controlled. If fact, in all probability, no single treatment will cure a patient with late-stage prostate cancer, but each successful clinical trial will provide doctors with another weapon in the arsenal of treatments for prostate cancer.

WHAT IS A CLINICAL TRIAL?

Simply put, clinical trials are research studies in which people help doctors find ways to improve cancer care. Each study poses a specific scientific question about how to prevent, diagnose, or treat cancer.

There are several types of clinical trials:

• *Prevention trials* test new approaches to reduce a person's risk of developing cancer. Most prevention trials are conducted on healthy people who have not had cancer. Some involve people who have had cancer and want to prevent recurrence, or people at higher risk than the general population.

• *Screening trials* test the best way to detect cancer, especially in its earliest stages. They are often conducted to determine whether a specific test used to detect cancer before it causes symptoms decreases the chance of dying from the disease. Examples in prostate cancer are the newer variations on the PSA blood test. These trials involve people who do not have any symptoms of cancer.

• *Diagnostic trials* study tests or procedures that could be used to identify cancer more accurately and at an early stage. Diagnostic trials usually include people who have signs or symptoms of cancer.

• *Treatment trials* are conducted with people who have cancer. They are designed to answer specific questions about, and evaluate the effectiveness of, a new treatment or a new way of using a standard treatment. These trials test many types of treatments, such as drugs, vaccines, new approaches to surgery or radiation therapy, or new combinations of treatments.

• *Quality-of-life trials* (also called supportive care trials) explore ways to improve comfort and quality of life for cancer patients. These trials may study ways to help people who are experiencing nausea, vomiting, sleep disorders, depression, or other effects from cancer or its treatment. Many treatment trials include quality-of-life assessments as well.

Clinical trials can be sponsored by government agencies, cooperative research groups, private drug and biotechnology companies, or even individual physicians. They may be conducted in university hospitals, medical centers, the National Cancer Institute (NCI), community hospitals, or even private doctors' offices. A study may take place at one or two locations or in dozens of centers nationwide, with results being submitted to a central location.

A man's doctor may recommend that he participate in a clinical trial, or the patient may learn about various studies in progress and raise the topic with his doctor. Whether the subject is raised by the patient or the doctor, it is essential that you openly discuss the topic with your health care provider to determine whether participating in a trial is right for you.

PROS AND CONS OF PARTICIPATING IN A TRIAL

Clinical trials by definition involve testing on human subjects. While every precaution is taken to prevent harmful side effects, patients may face some risk. Experts review and try to predict side effects, but it is impossible for researchers to identify every possible consequence of a new medicine or treatment. In fact, initial, or Phase I, trials have as their goal detecting the side effects and tolerability of a new drug or treatment as the dose is escalated. Before consenting to a trial, a patient and his family should be aware of all of the possible risks and benefits he faces by taking part in the research.

I believe that most patients who participate in clinical trials receive excellent individualized medical care and benefit from taking part in a trial, whether or not the agent being tested in the trial is proven to be effective. Patients in trials often receive ongoing treatment from three or four physicians as well as research nurses; in many studies, there are mandated treatment schedules that require full physical exams every three or four weeks. This high standard of care makes it much more likely that any health problems will be detected and corrected, including even previously undiagnosed conditions. A man in a prostate cancer study will have his PSA monitored, of course, but he may also have his blood pressure, liver and kidney functions, cholesterol levels, and other vital markers of overall health monitored at the same time. Some studies have found that people who participate in clinical trials tend to live longer than those with the same health profile who do not participate in research, even if the agent tested seems to have no effect. No doubt the excellence of health care and monitoring plays a role.

In many cases, patients in clinical trials have access to new therapies or medications that they wouldn't have been able to obtain if they weren't in the trial. Only rarely, however, do these medications offer lifesaving cures. Although desperate patients find hope in clinical trials, they should not consent with the expectation of a miraculous cure. A doctor suggesting a specific trial to a patient cannot promise a particular outcome, although it is likely that your participation will further medical knowledge about the treatment of prostate cancer.

Of course, not every trial is suitable for every patient. To qualify for a study, a man must meet the eligibility criteria, which typically involve his stage of cancer, previous treatments, and other health problems. Eligibility criteria are established prior to the initiation of a study. Even physicians involved in the trial cannot make exceptions to these criteria and permit the participation of a specific patient.

Only you can make the decision about whether or not to participate in a clinical trial. Before you make your decision, you should learn as much as possible about your disease and the trials available to you. Feel free to talk about this information with your doctor, family members, and friends to help you figure out whether or not a clinical trial is right for you.

In general, the potential benefits include:

- Your health care will be provided by physicians with expertise in prostate cancer treatment.

- You may receive access to new drugs and interventions before they are widely available.
- You will likely receive close monitoring of your health care and any side effects of the treatment.
- You will be able to take a more active role in your own health care.
- You may be one of the first to benefit from a new treatment.
- You will be able to make a contribution to the existing knowledge about the treatment of prostate cancer.

The potential risks include:

- New drugs and treatments may have side effects or risks unknown to the doctors. Although it is rare, a new agent can have unexpected, life-threatening consequences.
- New drugs and procedures may be ineffective or less effective than current treatments.
- Even if a new approach has benefits, it may not work for you.
- Often research trials involve more tests and office visits than routine care for the same condition.

HOW CLINICAL TRIALS ARE SUPPOSED TO WORK

Clinical trials must be conducted to prove a treatment's safety and efficacy, before the U.S. Food and Drug Administration will permit a medication to make its way into the market. Trials are conducted to evaluate new drugs as well as those that have been approved for use for another cancer or medical problem.

While the specific details vary from one trial to another, certain steps must be followed during any clinical trial. The following is a step-by-step summary of what takes place during a clinical trial.

Background Research and Protocol Design

Every trial begins with a hypothesis or a theory about why a new compound or procedure might be an effective treatment for prostate cancer or another disease. Researchers test these ideas in the laboratory and in animal studies. These preliminary studies give researchers clues about whether an experimental therapy will be helpful or harmful to humans.

If the treatment seems effective in animals, the researchers design a formal trial plan (also called a protocol) and submit an Investigational New Drug (IND) Application to the FDA. The protocol must undergo a scientific review to make sure that the scientific assumptions behind the study are sound enough to be approved by the FDA. Then both new drugs and new uses for existing drugs must be approved by local institutional review boards (IRBs) at the institution in which the trial will be performed. The IRB, which includes doctors, researchers, community leaders, and other members of the community, reviews the protocol to make sure the study is conducted fairly and participants are not likely to be harmed. The IRB can approve the trial as written, or it can determine that the protocol must be changed. In addition, the IRB has the power to stop a clinical trial if the researchers are not following the protocol or if the trial appears to be causing unexpected harm to the participants.

Not surprisingly, clinical trials have other layers of bureaucracy as well. Most larger or placebo-based trials must have a data and safety monitoring board (DSMB). The DSMB is an independent committee made up of statisticians, physicians, and other expert scientists, who monitor the data at regularly scheduled intervals. The DSMB can recommend that a trial be stopped if it recognizes that there is evidence to suggest that the risks of the trial outweigh the benefits. A DSMB can also stop a clinical trial if there is clear evidence that the new treatment is very effective, so that the beneficial treatment can be made widely available.

Before a clinical trial begins, the IRB reviews the patient consent forms and reviews the ethics of the trial. In addition, the IRB often will make sure that the primary researchers will not benefit financially from the research findings. Financial disclosure statements are required for every study. A researcher has a financial conflict of interest if he or she receives consulting income, gifts, or loans from the pharmaceutical company producing the drug, or if the researcher has investments in the firm or in a competing firm.

From a researcher's point of view, the best-designed clinical trials are prospective randomized studies, in which patients are put into two groups—one that will receive the test treatment and another that will receive standard therapy. In many cases, neither the patient nor the physician knows which treatment the patient is receiving. This is a double-blind trial. In a single-blind trial, the physician is aware of the specific treatment, but the patient is not. In situations in which there might not be any standard therapy for comparison, placebo-based trials might be instituted. As a rule, patients don't like participating in placebo-controlled studies because they don't want to take a chance on not receiving treatment. However, these studies produce the most reliable data with the least risk of researcher bias. Also some placebo-based trials have a so called cross-over design so that patients on the placebo have the opportunity to receive the test drug after a specified period.

Recruiting Patients

Every study has its eligibility criteria, or guidelines for who can participate. Generally, participants in a study share a type and stage of cancer, age, gender, and previous treatment history. The eligibility criteria are included in the study plan.

Patients join studies in one of two primary ways: either they are asked by their doctors to join a clinical trial, or the patient initiates the search and attempts to find an appropriate trial. In most cases, when placement is patient driven, it is because a patient has tried all of the traditional therapies without success and now seeks experimental treatments. These patients have typically gone through a series of treatments, from least toxic to most toxic. When one course of treatment fails, they move on to the next. When the range of common treatments fails, these patients turn to clinical trials in the hope of achieving a response.

Most studies have detailed criteria describing the types of patients appropriate for the specific study. Sometimes researchers may place ads in local newspapers or on Web sites to attract patients. In most cases, payments are not given in clinical trials for medical treatments or procedures, but participants may be reimbursed for transportation, parking, and other expenses.

It can be difficult to find the right patients for a trial. Researchers usually limit entry to patients who are otherwise healthy and do not have other health problems or second cancers. People with anemia, diabetes, or cardiovascular disease may not be eligible for a particular study. In addition, the researchers want to ensure that the patients will survive the course of the study, if at all possible, so that the results of treatment can be observed. Finally, because an investigative agent might be metabolized more slowly than expected, often normal kidney or liver capacity is required.

The search for the most appropriate patients must be balanced against the motivation of some researchers to recruit patients. Though your doctor may not tell you, sometimes researchers are compensated in some way for the number of patients they bring into a study; others feel pressure to conduct a number of studies and publish the results to further their professional goals.

The patient's individual needs should drive any decision about whether to participate in a trial. A patient should be able to ask the researcher, "Would you advise your father or brother or uncle to participate in this study if he had the same cancer history that I have?" If your doctor can't affirmatively recommend the trial to a loved one, he or she may have no business recommending it to a patient.

For almost all prostate cancer trials, you hopefully will not have to travel far from home to participate. Major hospitals, often within at least several hours' drive, typically will have a number of trials from which to choose. In addition, many trials, especially Phase III trials, are conducted in doctors' offices or multiple medical centers across the United States and Canada.

Do You *Really* Know What You're in For?

Doctors don't like surprises any more than their patients do. To keep participants in clinical trials fully informed of *everything* that will happen during the study, every patient must sign a detailed consent form before joining a trial.

Consent forms include details about the study

approach, the intervention given in the trial, the possible risks and benefits, and the tests you may have. The document helps demystify the research process, so that the patient has all the information he needs to decide if he would like to participate. These forms can be as long as thirty pages, but they are written in plain English. For example, rather than mentioning that the patient will donate 10cc of blood on a monthly basis, the form would say two teaspoons of blood. Any information that is not clear should be clarified by the doctor before a patient signs.

I encourage all my patients to take the consent form home and write any questions they might have in the margins. I ask them to underline any statement that they don't fully understand. When they bring the form back, we review every detail before signing the document. Sometimes patients are asked to initial each page to be sure they understand it. Some patients put their trust in the doctor and don't want to know the details. I appreciate the trust my patients have in me, but I want them to take responsibility for their health by reviewing the form anyway.

The consent form includes specific details on the trial itself, as well as details such as whether the patient will be reimbursed for parking expenses and who is responsible for medical care if the patient develops any complications during the trial. (Many health insurance companies refuse to cover medical problems that arise as a side effect of participation in a clinical trial. Instead, the cost of this care might shift to the pharmaceutical company sponsoring the trial.)

The consent form must be reissued during the study if the risks, benefits, or side effects change during the course of the research. For example, if a drug is shown to cause stroke in patients with cardiovascular disease, all participants (including those with no known history of cardio-vascular disease) will have to sign new forms acknowledging the potential risk. This process is designed to protect and inform patients.

Keep in mind that signing a consent form does not prevent you from suing the pharmaceutical company (if it is providing the test drug) or the medical facility if you experience complications due to negligence. Most IRBs will not permit consent forms to indemnify or protect the researchers from all lawsuits.

Signing a consent form also does not obligate you to remain in the study. You have the right to change your mind and leave the trial at any time. The consent form is designed to protect you, not to compel you to participate when you are longer interested.

Phase I Trials

Phase I trials evaluate how a new drug should be administered (by mouth, injected into the blood, or injected into the muscle), how often it should be given, and what dose is safe. Phase I studies, also known as safety studies, generally involve ten to one hundred healthy volunteers or patients and last for several months. The purposes of Phase I trials are to determine what is the maximum tolerated dose, what a safe dose is for patients, and what side effects might be expected. Also, sometimes the rates of metabolism of the test agent are assessed.

During this part of the trial, patients receive drugs at doses that range from ineffective to potentially excessive. The patients are divided into smaller groups, called cohorts. Each cohort is treated with an incremental dose of the new therapy or technique. The highest dose with an acceptable level of side effects is determined to be appropriate for further testing. About 70 percent of experimental drugs pass this initial phase of testing.

Many people who participate in Phase I trials do not understand why they are participating. Even when the risks and benefits are clearly spelled out in the consent forms, many patients do not understand that they may not benefit from a Phase I trial. In truth, only a small percentage of people in Phase I trials benefit directly from the drug they are testing. However, a 1995 University of Chicago study revealed that when asked about why they participated in a Phase I cancer trial, 85 percent of patients answered that they expected "possible therapeutic benefit."

Phase II Trials

Once a drug has been shown to be safe at a specific dose, it must be tested for efficacy. This second phase of testing may last from several months to years and often involves more than a hundred patients. Only about one-third of experimental drugs successfully complete both Phase I and Phase II studies. During Phase II trials, researchers may add a control group so they can look for signs that the therapy is having some effect.

Phase III Trials

Phase III trials test a new drug, a new combination of drugs, or a new surgical procedure in comparison to the current standard. A participant will be assigned randomly to either the new treatment or the standard treatment. In cases where there is no standard therapy, there might be a placebo arm of the trial. In some trials, there may be more than two arms or alternative therapies being tested.

Phase III studies involve several hundred to several thousand patients and may last for several years. About 80 percent of drugs that enter Phase III testing ultimately achieve FDA approval.

In treatment trials involving people with aggressive cancers, placebos (dummy pills that contain no active ingredient) are not commonly used. Instead, most studies are designed to compare a new treatment with a standard treatment. When no standard treatment exists, a study may compare a new treatment with a placebo, but you will be told about this possibility during the informed consent.

Phase IV

If a treatment proves safe and effective, the FDA approves the drug for widespread use. For up to ten years after approval, drug manufacturers are required to report to the FDA any unexpected adverse reactions caused by the drug.

Adverse events are listed by degree of severity: Grade 1 (minimal complaints that don't require medication), Grade 2 (minimal complaints that can be corrected with medication), Grade 3 (serious complaints that do not require hospitalization), Grade 4 (complications requiring hospitalization), and Grade 5 (death). Adverse events need to be reported to the pharmaceutical company during any phase (I through IV) of drug testing.

Doctors must report symptoms, even if they do not appear to be drug related. This reporting system allows doctors to recognize patterns of complications that might go unnoticed otherwise. A single event might seem unrelated to the use of a drug, but a cluster of similar complaints may indicate a side effect that may be linked to the medication.

QUESTIONS TO ASK BEFORE JOINING A TRIAL

Before agreeing to participate in a clinical trial, you should have a frank discussion with your doctor. Consider taking a family member or friend along to the doctor's office for support and to help get all your questions answered.

Write down all your questions in advance; write down the answers so that you can review them. If you feel more comfortable, consider bringing a tape recorder so that you can review the doctor's responses after the appointment, if necessary. Be sure to cover the following questions:

About the Study

- What is the primary purpose of the clinical trial? What is the specific treatment being evaluated, or in what way will this trial advance medical knowledge?
- Who is sponsoring the trial? The federal government? A private drug or biotechnology company? (Some patients feel more comfortable participating in a National Cancer Institute–sponsored trial, instead of one funded by a pharmaceutical company.)
- Why do researchers think the experimental approach may be effective?
- What is already known about the drug?
- What phase is the trial—I, II, or III? (The earlier the phase, the more experimental the procedure or treatment.)
- Who has reviewed and approved the study?
- How are the study results and safety of participants being checked?

- How long will the study last?
- Can I drop out of the study if I change my mind?
- What will my responsibilities be if I participate?
- Can I continue to take all my current medications?
- Can I take nutritional supplements or herbs?
- Will I be able to see my regular doctor? When do I see the study doctors?
- Where else is this study being performed?

Possible Risks and Benefits

- How will I benefit from my participation? (You may choose to participate in a study even if you will not personally benefit because it will advance medical knowledge about prostate cancer.)
- What are my possible short-term risks?
- What are my possible long-term risks?
- What other options do people with my cancer history have?
- How do the possible risks and benefits of this trial compare with those options?
- If the research is already under way, can you provide a synopsis of how the other patients have tolerated the treatment up to this point? (The research physician may not be allowed to know these results, however.)
- How many other patients have received the drug or treatment in this trial or in previous trials? What are the experiences to date?

What to Expect

- What kinds of therapies, procedures, and tests will I have during the trial?

- How do the tests in the study compare with those I would have outside the trial?
- Where will I receive my medical care?
- Who will be in charge of my care?
- What is the track record of the primary investigator? How long has he or she been conducting trials?
- What procedures will I follow to report any problems or sudden changes during the study? Is the contact person available twenty-four hours a day by cell phone or pager?

Personal Concerns

- How could being in this study affect my daily life?
- Can I talk to other people in the study?
- How much time will it take for me to participate in this study?

Cost Concerns

- Will I have to pay for any part of the trial, such as tests or the study drug? If so, what will the charges be?
- What is my health insurance likely to cover?
- Who can help answer any questions from my insurance company or health plan?
- Will there be any travel or child care costs that I need to consider while I am in the trial?

A Tainted Past

When joining a clinical trial, some patients joke that they are signing on to serve as human guinea pigs. Our job as clinical investigators and medical professionals is to ensure that every patient participating in a trial understands the potential risks and benefits of the research, and we must do all that we can to minimize any possible harm. Despite some recent well-publicized cases of complications that occurred during clinical trials, I believe that it has never been safer than it is today to participate in one.

Unfortunately, doctors have not always followed the highest ethical standards when designing their research projects. Before 1974, researchers and their financial supporters were free to decide what constituted ethical research. Most researchers exercised sound judgment, but a few appalling examples of abuse stand out.

A few chilling stories:

- In the 1930s, doctors at the Tuskegee Institute in Georgia withheld treatment from African Americans with syphilis so that they could monitor the progression of the disease.
- In the 1950s, the U.S. Army gave LSD to soldiers without their knowledge or consent.
- In the 1950s, mentally retarded children at a state institution in New York were intentionally infected with hepatitis so that researchers could work on an experimental vaccine.
- In the 1960s, researchers injected prisoners and terminally ill patients with live cancer cells to test their immune responses.

In response to such abuses, Congress passed the National Research Act of 1974, which required the formation of institutional review boards to approve and monitor all federally funded research. (As a matter of practice, private research follows the same standards as well.) The Department of Health and Human Services has since created the Office for Human Research Protection, which supervises and monitors the review boards.

While I support such protections, the burden of paperwork has become quite daunting. This bureaucracy enhances safety, but it increases the cost of research. In some cases, the process has become so slow and cumbersome that it has delayed important research.

The bottom line: Clinicians are forced to walk an ethical and scientific tightrope. If the rules protecting patients are too lax, subjects will suffer and perhaps die. On the other hand, if the rules are too strict, lifesaving medications won't make it out of the laboratory quickly enough to help the people who need them most.

OTHER WAYS TO GET EXPERIMENTAL DRUGS

Most patients must participate in clinical trials in order to obtain drugs that have not been approved by the FDA. Some, however, may receive investigational drugs through an expanded access protocol or by a mechanism known as a special or compassionate exception.

Expanded access. Expanded access protocols are available for a limited number of investigational drugs that have been well studied and are awaiting final FDA approval for marketing. Expanded access allows a wider group of people to be treated with the drug. The purpose of an expanded access program is to make investigational drugs that have significant activity against specific cancers available to patients before the FDA approval process has been completed.

The drug company or sponsor must apply to the FDA to

make the drug available through an expanded access program. There must be enough evidence from the studies to show that the drug may be effective to treat a specific type of cancer without unreasonable risks. The FDA generally approves expanded access only if there are no other satisfactory treatments available for the disease. It's important to note that patients still need to qualify for these studies. Some patients with liver or kidney problems might not be able to participate.

Compassionate exemption. Patients who do not meet the eligibility criteria for a clinical trial of an investigational drug may be eligible to receive the drug under a provision known as a compassionate exemption or compassionate use. The patient's doctor contacts the sponsor of the clinical trial and provides the patient's medical information and treatment history. Requests are evaluated on a case-by-case basis. The FDA often must approve each request. There should be reasonable expectation that the drug will prolong a patient's life or improve quality of life. In some cases, even patients who qualify for treatment with an investigational drug on a compassionate basis might not be able to obtain it if the drug is in limited supply. In prostate cancer therapy, it is often difficult to get investigational drugs through expanded access or compassionate use.

Who Pays Your Medical Expenses?

Many health insurance and managed care providers refuse to cover the patient care costs associated with a clinical trial if a drug is considered investigational or experimental. (Some will cover expenses once a treatment is established as safe and effective.) Before agreeing to participate in a study, you may want to ask someone from the research team to talk to your health insurance plan to clarify your possible coverage.

Some states have passed legislation that requires health insurers to cover the costs of certain trials. For more information, visit the National Cancer Institute's state initiatives and legislation digest page at http://cancer.gov/clinicaltrials/insurancelaws on the Internet.

Many federal health care programs do pay the cost of coverage:

- Medicare covers costs for beneficiaries who participate in clinical trials designed to diagnose or treat cancer. For more information, call l-800-MEDICARE or visit the Web site http://medicare.gov.
- TRICARE, the Department of Defense's health program, reimburses beneficiaries for costs associated with participation in a National Cancer Institute–sponsored Phase II or Phase III cancer prevention (including screening and early detection) or treatment trial. For more information, visit http://cis.nci.nih.gov/fact/1_13.htm.
- The Department of Veterans Affairs (VA) covers costs of veterans who participate in NCI-sponsored prevention, diagnosis, and treatment studies. For more information, visit http://cis.nci.gov/fact/1_17.htm.

FINDING A CLINICAL TRIAL

If you do want to participate in a clinical trial, start by discussing the matter with your doctor. The idea of participating in a trial may originate with the doctor or a patient. Most doctors will make referrals to appropriate studies if they believe a patient is suitable for one. In some cases, doctors won't make referrals because they believe a patient is too sick to be a good participant.

Your doctor does not need to be a genitourinary oncologist to recommend appropriate trials for men with prostate cancer. Such specialists tend to work in academic settings, but general oncologists often know a considerable amount about clinical trials going on in their areas. More than ten thousand physicians in the United States and Canada take part in trials sponsored by the National Cancer Institute.

You can also do research on your own to find out which studies are available. Survivor networks and prostate cancer support groups can be an excellent resource. (See chapter 12 for information on finding support groups.) Many of these groups can offer specific contact information and personal anecdotal information about ongoing research.

If you're a discriminating researcher, you can find a great deal of information about clinical trials by using the Internet. In fact, I receive e-mails every week from people who want more information about various clinical trials in progress.

You cannot enroll for a clinical trial online. In most cases, you can call a research nurse, who will interview you to determine if you fit the profile of patients appropriate for the trial. Always be truthful when describing your medical history; the researchers will obtain copies of your medical records when screening you for the trial.

The following Web sites often list hundreds of ongoing trials. Each study description includes the medical profile of men who are appropriate candidates. For example, a clinical trial may call for men with prostate cancer who have not received radiation therapy, or patients who have already had one chemotherapy regimen. Follow up with a call to the researchers only if you meet the stated study guidelines.

• *www.cancer.gov* The National Cancer Institute is a component of the National Institutes of Health, one of the eight agencies that compose the Public Health Service in the Department of Health and Human Services. NCI is the federal government's principal agency for cancer research and training. The institute's comprehensive site is great for finding cancer trials and keeping track of cancer research results. The most exhaustive database of cancer clinical trials is the National Cancer Institute's PDQ database, accessible through the NCI Web site. PDQ includes most trials sponsored or conducted by NCI. It also includes many cancer trials sponsored by pharmaceutical companies, medical centers, and other groups. It lists both active studies (currently enrolling patients) and those closed to enrollment. You can also make online requests for a wide range of publications and booklets designed for cancer patients, health care professionals, and the general public. Many are offered in both English and Spanish.

• *www.Acurian.com* This Web site, which is designed to accelerate clinical trial recruitment for pharmaceutical and biotechnology companies, lists clinical trials currently enrolling patients. It also includes information on drugs in development and news from medical and research resources.

• *www.acs.org* The American Cancer Society supported forty-nine clinical research projects in 2000, including twelve early (Phase I or II) clinical trials. General information on ACS research is available from its Web site and by calling 800-ACS-2345. The site includes information about cancers, treatment options, and clinical trials.

• *www.prostatecancerfoundation.org* The Prostate Cancer Foundation is dedicated to research and education on prostate cancer. At this writing, the foundation is sponsoring more than sixty clinical trials in twelve locations around the country. For more information, including a list of trials, call 800-757-CURE.

• *www.centerwatch.com* CenterWatch is a Boston-based company that provides patients with a variety of information about clinical trials. This Web site lists more than forty-one thousand industry- and government-sponsored clinical trials as well as new drug therapies recently approved by the FDA. Check out *Informed Consent,* a book sold through the site, which provides advice to patients participating in trials.

Call for Help

Cancer Treatment Consultants is an organization that helps cancer patients and their families sift through the treatment options and find a prostate cancer clinical trial that may be appropriate. You can search for prostate cancer clinical trials on this site by simply following the four-step process outlined in the clinical trials section. For more information, visit the Web site http:www.411cancer.com.

Chapter 8

◦◦◦

Considering Your Options: Choosing the Best Treatment Plan for You

Most of the time when we speak of life-or-death decisions, we speak in hyperbole. In life, we rarely confront such monumental choices; for most of us, destiny doesn't boil down to a single question. But men who are diagnosed with prostate cancer often feel that they must consider their options for treatment as if there is a single "right" course of treatment that they must identify from a confusing array of options. It is something of a tragedy that patients often feel as if their lives depend on this decision, because most often this is not the case.

Prostate cancer is different from most other cancers because in general, there is no exact standard of care for the disease at its different stages. There has not been sufficient research for us to determine with certainty if one treatment method is preferable to another in the treatment of most cases of early prostate cancer. Therefore, most often men with the disease feel the burden of choosing the type of treatment they receive.

For individual patients, the decision often involves trade-offs in the risks of lifestyle changes and side effects. What role does potency play in your life? How would you cope if you developed permanent incontinence?

I tell my patients not to feel that they have their fate in their hands, but they do have choices to make about the possible risks they will have to accept with different treatments. Most important, there is no need to rush into a specific treatment. In most cases, a patient will have weeks to decide on a course of therapy.

I wish I had a crystal ball so that I could see the future and tell men which treatment would be most effective, and which side effects would have the greatest impact on their lives. Unfortunately, I do not. And so the best I can do is explain the decision-making process and reassure my patients that the decision is not one of life or death. Most often it is the biology of the cancer that will determine the outcome of the disease, not the patient's choice of treatment.

NO CLEAR ANSWERS

Ideally, researchers studying prostate cancer would have been able to compare the efficacy of one treatment option with another, similar to what has been done for women with breast cancer. Studies have randomly assigned women to treatment via radiation and lumpectomy (removal of a portion of breast tissue) or mastectomy (removal of the entire breast). With a couple of exceptions, oncologists now tell women and their spouses that lumpectomy is a recommended treatment with no statistically greater risk of relapse and a better cosmetic outcome. These women have a database to guide this decision.

Why haven't we done this type of prospective randomized trial for prostate cancer? Because it's difficult to randomly assign patients into such radically different therapies. Researchers can do retrospective analyses, which assess the patient's treatment and outcome, but this approach does not control for selection of the patients.

Another problem with comparing therapies is that both radiation and surgery treatments have changed dramatically over time. For example, complex computer programs constantly improve the ability of radiation oncologists to focus the radiation on the prostate and spare the rectum and bladder, and surgeons often refine and improve their techniques to spare the nerves and avoid incontinence. This progress is reassuring to the patient, but it makes it difficult to design an accurate study to compare approaches.

PREDICTING THE EXTENT OF YOUR PROSTATE CANCER

Learning that you have prostate cancer will open you to a range of follow-up questions. One of the most important is: *Has my cancer spread beyond the prostate?*

Doctors look at several variables to assess the likelihood that the cancer has spread. These include the PSA level, the Gleason score, and the clinical stage (what the cancer feels like during a digital rectal exam). Using these factors, researchers at Johns Hopkins University designed the Partin tables, which determine the *probability* that the cancer has spread.

These tables don't predict whether or not you will be cured with surgery or any form of radiation therapy, but they do list averages for whether the cancer has moved outside the gland itself. The numbers have a 95 percent confidence interval, meaning they will be accurate ninety-five times out of a hundred. This information may play a critical role in the treatment you choose. (For example, surgery is not recommended if the cancer has spread beyond the prostate.) For a simplified version of the Partin tables, see Appendix B.

MAKING SENSE OF THE NUMBERS

The Partin tables may help you understand the likelihood that your cancer has moved beyond the prostate. Using that information, as well as other characteristics of your cancer, you must face a decision about what treatment to follow.

In addition to the Partin tables, physicians who care for prostate cancer patients have a system of assessing risk for relapse after primary therapy, or progression for those men who choose the watchful waiting approach. We categorize prostate cancer into good-risk, intermediate-risk, and high-risk groups:

- Good-risk patients have T1c or T2a disease, PSA levels of less than or equal to 10, and a Gleason score of 6 or less.
- Intermediate-risk patients have stage T2b disease, PSA levels between 10 and 20, and a Gleason score of 7. We also weigh the impact of the frequency with which the core biopsies exhibited cancer in this risk group. To be classified as intermediate disease, less than one-third of the cores in a biopsy should show cancer.
- High-risk patients are those with T2c disease or higher, PSA levels over 20, Gleason scores of 8 or above, or more than 34 percent of the core biopsies showing cancer.

Any of the higher-risk features increases the risk to the next group. For example, if a patient has T1c stage disease, a PSA level less than 10, only one of six cores showing cancer, but a Gleason pattern of 8 or more, he would be classified as high risk. Still, in situations such as this where there is an apparent disparity among risk factors, it might be prudent to have the pathology of the core biopsies examined at another institution. You can request that your pathology slides be sent to commercial laboratories. (Ask your doctor for a recommendation.)

Also, if you decide to seek a second opinion about your cancer, consider obtaining one from a different institution or office than where you sought your first opinion. In this case, the pathology slides will often be assessed by a different pathologist, and you can ask if the reading was the same. One more caveat about using this risk system: Although PSA levels are affected by the amount of cancer in your body, before primary therapy these levels are also affected by the size of your prostate gland (as discussed in chapter 1). Therefore, it is possible that a patient with a large prostate gland (more than a hundred grams) could have a PSA level over 10 and be classified as low risk if he had other low-risk characteristics.

If you fall into the intermediate- or high-risk category, you will probably undergo a series of tests to further stage the disease. Among the tests that might be ordered are a bone scan, a CT scan of the abdomen or pelvis, and an endorectal MRI, or magnetic resonance imaging. All of these tests have a possible false negative rate—they don't always detect cancer when it is actually present. The CT scan and bone scan are performed to determine if the disease had metastasized. The MRI may be performed to determine if the disease has invaded the prostate capsule. Still, these tests are critical, and have the highest rate of detecting cancer in patients with high-risk features. Many physicians don't order these tests for patients with low-risk features of the disease, and I don't believe they are necessary for those patients.

In this chapter, I have discussed different features of prostate cancer. This has been done to guide you when discussing your case with others. So often a patient will tell me that a friend had prostate cancer and was told he could watch it or that he was a good candidate for external-beam radiation or another therapy. Now my patient wants to know why his prostate cancer cannot be treated in the same way. It is essential to remember that prostate cancer has a wide spectrum of risk. In a sense, it is really many different kinds of disease with some common features. Be careful when extrapolating another person's experience to your own.

Now that we have discussed the general risk categories for prostate cancer and the risk for spread outside the gland, we can begin to make headway in understanding what kind of therapy might be best for you. In general:

- If you have low-risk features, you are a candidate for surgery, brachytherapy, or in some cases watchful waiting.
- If you have intermediate-risk features, you are a candidate for surgery, external-beam radiation therapy, with or without neoadjuvant hormone therapy (see page 73), and sometimes brachytherapy alone or with external-beam therapy.
- If you have high-risk features, it is important to consider some forms of combined therapies; often, a single form of primary therapy is insufficient. Many patients are currently treated with external-beam radiation and neoadjuvant hormonal therapy.

IS WATCHFUL WAITING RIGHT FOR YOU?

Not everyone needs primary therapy right away. Researchers haven't established criteria for men who are good candidates for watchful waiting. In the future, molecular markers might help us with this problem so that we can better categorize risk for progression compared to the tools we now have. However, you might consider watchful waiting if:

- You have a PSA of 4.0 or less; or a PSA density below 0.1 or 0.15.
- There are no abnormalities in a digital rectal exam.
- You have a low Gleason score (6 or less).
- You have a very low prostate volume (one out of twelve cores on a biopsy positive, and a small percentage of that core is involved).

Age is another important variable. In general, if you're seventy-five or older and have low-risk disease, you might not need primary treatment. At age eighty, even moderate-risk disease may not need intervention. At eighty-five and older, there is often little need for any form of primary treatment.

On the other hand, I do not routinely recommend watchful waiting for most men in their forties, fifties, or early sixties. The disease will likely progress, and younger men have decades of additional risk ahead. The problem with following patients for a long period is that we don't have reliable methods for determining progression. As I've noted, we don't really know how to do the "watch" part of watchful waiting. In the coming years, men may be able to have their condition monitored using a modification of an existing test, such as the endorectal (in the anus) MRI. Using this technique, doctors may be able to monitor the progression of the disease, recommending treatment only when the cancer begins to grow. In this way, a man could avoid the side effects of treatment until absolutely necessary. As I stated before, however, this method is not capable yet of reliably monitoring progression within the prostate gland.

Any man choosing watchful waiting should have his PSA

checked every three to six months, and he should be aware that the cancer can progress even if the PSA level does not rise. A study conducted in Finland found that men who choose watchful waiting died twice as often from prostate cancer as those who opted for primary therapy. However, these men had more advanced prostate cancer than those we detect routinely in the United States.

TREATING LOCAL PROSTATE CANCER

Prostate cancer restricted to the gland itself is referred to as local cancer. This is the stage of disease overwhelmingly diagnosed currently in the United States. In addition to taking into account factors about the cancer, consider factors regarding your own health when deciding between radiation therapies and surgery. Additional factors to consider:

• Men with severe heart disease, heart arrhythmia, or bleeding disorders should avoid surgery, if possible. If a man with cardiovascular problems is debating between surgery and radiation, he may opt for the radiation therapy to avoid the possible complications of the anesthesia and the surgical procedure.

• The risk of surgery increases in men as they age. Older men experience a greater risk of complications from anesthesia, as well as a higher level of postoperative complications.

• Men with ulcerative colitis of the rectum, chronic diarrhea, or other bowel disease should consider avoiding all types of radiation therapy, especially external-beam radiation therapy. The radiation may damage the rectum or colon, exacerbating the digestive problems.

• Brachytherapy (seed radiation therapy) should probably be used only by men with a Gleason score below 7 (3 + 4).

Brachytherapy is as good as external-beam radiation in men who do not have large prostate nodules, and when the gland is not too large. Patients with intermediate- or high-risk features have a high rate of relapse if treated with brachytherapy alone.

GUIDELINES FOR ADVANCED LOCAL PROSTATE CANCER

What should you do if you have intermediate- or high-risk features of the disease? You may benefit from more than one form of therapy. For example, there is evidence that patients with high-risk features do better if they receive hormonal therapy in conjunction with external-beam radiation therapy. The hormonal therapy is typically initiated a few months prior to the radiation therapy; this is called neoadjuvant therapy. The hormones can also be administered at the same time as the radiation therapy, a procedure known as adjuvant therapy. We don't know if one approach is preferable to another. This combination approach helps address the minimal residual disease that may be present outside the gland, or, more likely, it may aid the radiation in treating local cancer. It is unusual that a man with high-risk features would be treated with either hormones or surgery and radiation alone.

There are other forms of combined therapy for high-risk patients. Some physicians recommend combining brachytherapy with external-beam radiation. In this approach, men receive about two-thirds of the typical dose of external therapy and brachytherapy, in either order. The overall external-beam radiation dose is limited to spare patients some of the side effects associated with full-dose radiation therapy. The external-beam therapy is important for patients with some risk and a disease that may have spread microscopically outside the prostate.

Another form of combination therapy is treatment with

external-beam radiation several months after surgery. This might be recommended more frequently to a patient whose prostate gland has a positive margin, meaning the cancer has been "cut through" by the surgeon's scalpel at the location of a tumor but there are still cancer cells at the edge of the tissue that was removed. We don't know if this is necessary in every case; it might depend on where within the prostate gland the positive margin was detected. In any case, radiation therapy should not be administered until the patient is fully continent. Radiation therapy tends to inhibit healing, and might render a patient incontinent if administered too soon after surgery. It is not yet known if the adjuvant form of radiation therapy provides a survival advantage to patients.

SALVAGE THERAPY: IF PSA RISES AFTER PRIMARY THERAPY

After treatment, every man prays that his cancer will be gone—forever. Unfortunately, some 30 to 40 percent of men will experience a recurrence of cancer at some point during their lifetimes. In almost every case, the recurrence is first diagnosed by rising PSA levels. Patients often are tested every six months, although there is no standard. After surgery, a man's PSA should drop to an undetectable level. After radiation, the level should drop below 1.0. If the level is higher than these thresholds after treatment, the patient has a high risk for relapse. Most recurrences occur within the first five years of the primary treatment. Still, even if the PSA starts rising after surgery or radiation therapy, many patients will remain clinically free of symptoms for extended periods of time, typically measured in years.

Should a patient's PSA level rise after surgery or radiation therapy, it is important to establish the PSA doubling time (as described in chapter 2). This is the number of months it would take for a man's PSA level to climb, for example, from 1.5 to 3.0. If the PSA doubling time is relatively long (more than one year), it can be predicted that it will take a relatively long time for the cancer to show up as metastases in other sites in the body. If, on the other hand, the doubling time is short (three months or less), it can be predicted that it will take a relatively short time for the cancer to spread. On average, if a man has a doubling time of ten months, it will be about eight years from the time his PSA rises to the time the cancer is evident in a distant site such as his bones. These observations are documented in an article published in the *Journal of the American Medical Association* in 1999.

The median age at the time of diagnosis is seventy-two years. If the cancer recurs, a man may undergo secondary or salvage therapy. These treatments can continue to extend his natural life by controlling the progression of the disease. There is no standard of care for salvage therapy. The treatment choices depend, in part, on the type of primary therapy a man previously chose. The following are some guidelines for salvage treatment.

If a man has had a radical prostatectomy, he can have salvage radiation therapy, with moderate or minimal risk of side effects. Salvage radiation therapy is considered successful when it results in PSA levels that decrease and don't rise again—but this happens in only about 20 percent of patients. When the procedure is unsuccessful, it is presumed that at the time of the salvage radiation, the cancer had already spread outside the radiation field to other sites in the body. Frequently the PSA drops after salvage radiation, only to increase again. This suggests that the patient had some, but not all, of his cancer within the pelvis.

If a man had primary radiation therapy, he cannot have a

routine radical prostatectomy as a salvage therapy because the surgery is likely to result in serious complications due to the buildup of scar tissue. Many men choose surgery over forms of radiation therapy because they will be eligible for salvage radiation therapy should their PSA levels rise after surgery. Although patients can safely receive salvage radiation therapy, it is not clear to me how much this factor should influence their decision making when choosing between surgery and radiation therapy. Remember that salvage radiation therapy in this setting is infrequently curative. This form of salvage radiation should be distinguished from adjuvant radiation therapy (radiation therapy given a few months after surgery for positive margins, as described above).

One of the largest groups of patients with prostate cancer in the United States is men with rising PSA levels after primary therapy who do not have any signs of metastatic disease. These patients face difficult treatment decisions. If they had a prostatectomy, they are eligible for salvage radiation therapy, but, as discussed above, even with this treatment the PSA levels often continue to rise after the radiation is completed.

These men are candidates for hormonal therapy, but we don't yet know whether hormonal therapy administered for a PSA rise only is a better form of treatment than waiting until a patient has signs of metastasis. Although it might make sense to treat a patient when his tumor burden is smaller, the duration of effectiveness of these therapies is limited. Furthermore, hormonal therapy has significant side effects (as described in chapter 5). Some data suggest that earlier treatment with hormonal therapy might result in longer survival, but because of the side effects, some physicians elect to treat with intermittent hormonal therapy to extend the time period that men can use these treatments. Treatment with hormone therapy for rising PSA levels should be distinguished from hormone therapy for symptomatic, metastatic disease. In this case, if a patient has not been treated with hormonal therapy, it is often the treatment of choice.

EXPERIMENTAL TREATMENTS: KEEPING CANCER AT BAY

Since hormone therapy is limited in its duration of effectiveness, many patients opt for experimental therapies that *might* prolong their PSA doubling times. These treatments will not cure the cancer, but if they can slow the doubling time, it might delay the need for hormone therapy. Some of the experimental treatment for patients with rising PSA levels but no signs of metastasis include vaccine therapy, COX-2 inhibitors, and even the use of herbs and nutritional supplements.

This chapter has summarized the factors that a man should consider when choosing a course of treatment for his prostate cancer. The following chapter describes how herbs and nutritional supplements can be used to prevent or slow the recurrence of prostate cancer and to treat benign prostate problems.

Chapter 9

—◦∞◦—

Natural Remedies:
The Wise Use of Herbs and
Nutritional Supplements

Cancer is a bully. It preys on the vulnerable, especially those who are genetically predisposed to be susceptible to the disease. There is also emerging evidence that a poor diet, lack of exercise, and other lifestyle choices may make cancers more aggressive. When it comes to prostate cancer, researchers suspect that there is no single genetic trigger that allows the cancer to take hold and spread. Instead, many factors play a role in determining how aggressive the disease will be in any single patient, including the genetic makeup of the cancer and the patient's own immune system.

There are some things patients can do to decrease the chances of prostate cancer gaining a foothold in the body. For instance, some herbs and nutritional supplements are now being tested for their role in prostate cancer prevention—and many of these appear to be safe. While I do not prescribe natural remedies as the first line of therapy for prostate cancer, I think they will be shown to play a role in the prevention of prostate cancer.

Most doctors are too dismissive of "natural treatments," but they would do well to remember the PC-SPES experience (see chapter 6). Natural treatments are unlikely to be curative in their own right—a patient with advanced cancer is very unlikely to become cancer-free by relying on products from the local health food store—but some evidence suggests that the natural remedies discussed in this chapter may help fight prostate cancer in its earliest stages or help prevent the disease. In addition, the evidence is quite strong that many herbs and nutritional supplements can help treat BPH and other benign prostate conditions.

In my experience, patients themselves are pushing mainstream doctors toward acceptance of natural remedies. Many of my patients collect information from the Internet and from books and magazines, and they want to try every remedy available to them. Too many physicians fail to recognize the potential importance these remedies have to patients. It's critical that doctors be open to discussions about these remedies with their patients, sharing the information that is known about them, admitting the many gaps in medical knowledge about their use and efficacy, and sometimes warning patients about their possible unknown side effects.

Doctors need to talk about these remedies because their patients *are* going to use them, whether or not they tell their doctor about it. Problems can arise when certain natural, over-the-counter treatments interact with prescription drugs, causing unwanted side effects or altering the results of various diagnostic tests. These harmful interactions are more likely to be avoided if the primary physician is familiar with *all* medications—prescription, over-the-counter, and herbal—that the patient is taking.

While I support research on natural remedies, I approach the subject with a dose of skepticism. When it comes to natural remedies, physicians and patients need to be critical consumers of medical information. Don't trust anecdotal information posted on the Internet and many of the claims of infomercials. There are snake oil salesmen peddling false hope in the form of "cures" for every kind of cancer, including prostate cancer. These claims make it difficult for both doctors and patients to determine which have merit. Research has been conducted on some of these products, and other studies are now under way, but there are too many products for the research establishment to study. My motto: Be open-minded, but skeptical.

Toward that end, patients and physicians need to remember that they are partners in the healing process. They need to work together to share information about natural treatments—or any other matter—with respect and openness. You as a patient need to feel comfortable discussing the use of herbs and supplements with your doctor. Sometimes this can be difficult, based on the personalities involved. Some patients are acutely interested in their treatment and want to understand every step, while others want to find a physician they trust and put their health care in that person's hands. I treat both types of patients, but in either case, the patient must feel comfortable communicating with his caretaker, especially about any medicine, supplement, or herb he is taking.

Another Way That Natural Remedies Heal

Too many of the patients I see have the false belief that their prostate cancer was somehow caused by something they did or something they failed to do. Was the cancer caused by too many fast-food meals? By the pack-a-day cigarette habit you've tried to kick for the past decade? Or maybe the cancer grew stronger as you grew weaker because you haven't exercised regularly since your days in Little League?

I try to reassure my patients that cancer happens to good people, and to fit and otherwise healthy people, too. Prostate cancer is not your fault. I find that many men benefit from taking some control of their health care. They need to do *something* to help their bodies confront the cancer, and taking medically proven herbs and natural remedies can be an appropriate step in some cases. But just as you didn't cause your prostate cancer by an unhealthy lifestyle, it might not be possible to reverse your cancer now by adopting a different diet or healthier lifestyle.

HERBAL TREATMENTS

Herbs and plants have been used in the treatment of disease for thousands of years. Medical historians tell us that the ancient Egyptians, Indians, and Chinese extensively used herbal remedies for a wide variety of disorders, including those affecting the prostate. In fact, historical records dating from 3000 B.C. show that Chinese physicians routinely used herbs for urinary frequency and other prostate-related symptoms.

Herbal medicine is one of the most popular forms of natural medicine today. Recent polls show, for example, that people are increasingly turning to herbs for the relief of many acute and chronic conditions. In some cases, this interest is well grounded—scientific evidence is now validating the many benefits of herbal medicine. Other times, however, well-done studies show no benefit to using an herbal remedy long thought to be effective. One example of this is echinacea; although widely touted as a cure for the common cold, there is little evidence of its utility. Many such claims are made for specific herbs and herbal preparations, but it is hard to double-check the facts.

HOW TO PURCHASE, PREPARE, AND USE HERBS

Herbs and herbal preparations are widely available at pharmacies, health food stores, and grocery stores. They typically come in capsule or liquid form. Loose herbs may also be purchased from shops that specialize in herbs. In some cases, they should be protected from sunlight and should not be stored in clear plastic bags.

It is essential to understand how herbs are administered. Traditionally, herbal administrations include the following:

• *Decoctions.* The hardiest parts of the herb, including its roots and bark, are boiled in water for ten minutes and then allowed to steep. One ounce of herbal material is added to 4 cups of water. If more than one herb is being used, the sum of the herbs should still equal 1 ounce. After straining the decoction, you drink it like a tea.

• *Infusions.* Boiling water is poured over the petals, flowers, or leaves of an herb, which then steep for twenty or more minutes. After straining the infusion, you drink it. Infusions are weaker than decoctions.

• *Tinctures.* Alcohol is used to extract the medicinal properties of an herb. One ounce of dried herbal material (or 3 ounces of fresh herbs) is mixed with 5 ounces of alcohol (hundred-proof vodka can be used). This preparation is then kept in a small, sterile, airtight bottle and allowed to stand for two to six weeks. Usually 1 or more teaspoons of the tincture are taken daily, unless otherwise prescribed. Tinctures are available at many health food stores.

• *Extracts.* Extracts are prepared like tinctures, except water is used as the extraction medium. If you plan on making your own extracts, remember that some herbs are better activated by preparing them in alcohol; if you have any questions on this matter, seek the help of a qualified herbalist, or purchase your extracts from a reputable health food store.

• *Capsules.* You can usually purchase any herb you wish in capsule form (capsules typically contain a pure concentration of finely ground dried herbs). If you use herbs, I recommend capsules standardized for particular active ingredients.

In order to make sure your herbs and nutritional supplements remain stable, they should be stored properly. Do not put them in the refrigerator or store them in the bathroom; they will be too moist. Keep them in a cupboard out of direct sunlight.

Saw Palmetto

For the first half of the twentieth century, American doctors prescribed saw palmetto for a number of disorders, including urinary frequency and prostatitis. In fact, saw palmetto was officially listed in the U.S. Pharmacopoeia and the National Formulary until 1950, when the U.S. Food and Drug Administration reclassified it as an unproven drug and removed it from the list. While the herb fell out of favor in the United States, it has consistently been used in Europe for the treatment of prostate disease. In Europe, it is sold as Permixon, a highly purified form of the plant extract.

There have been several well-performed double-blind trials evaluating saw palmetto. In these studies, saw palmetto was found to cause a statistically significant improvement in symptoms among men suffering from BPH. Additional studies have shown that saw palmetto also, like finasteride and dutasteride, weakly inhibits 5-alpha reductase and the production of dihydrotestosterone (DHT)—the by-product of testosterone that may have a stronger effect on prostate growth than testosterone. Extracts of saw palmetto have also been found to prevent DHT from binding to prostate cells. At present, researchers have not examined the impact of saw palmetto on the treatment or prevention of prostate cancer, but it does appear to have some benefit for BPH. Consider the evidence:

• According to an article reported in the March 2003 issue of *American Family Physician,* saw palmetto had effects similar to those of the medication finasteride, and it was better tolerated and less expensive. It was found to have no known drug interactions, and side effects are both minor and rare.

• A Russian study reported in the November 2002 issue of *Scientific Research Institute of Urology* involved 155 men with BPH who took 160 milligrams twice a day of Permixon (an extract of saw palmetto) for two years. While the men did not have a change in their PSA levels, they showed a significant improvement in BPH symptoms within six months. The authors concluded that saw palmetto should be the first-line treatment of BPH.

• An article in the May 2000 issue of the journal *Urology* reviewed literature and found that saw palmetto may have significant effects on urinary flow rates and symptom scores compared to placebo in men with lower urinary tract symptoms of BPH.

• Saw palmetto may also affect hormone levels in the prostate. A May 2001 article reported in the journal *Urology* found that a saw palmetto herbal blend caused a modest but significant suppression of dihydrotestosterone levels in a randomized trial.

How to take it. The components of saw palmetto that benefit the prostate are called liposterolic extracts, and they are mainly contained in the plant's berries. The berries are also rich in carotenes, polysaccharides, and fatty acids. When taking saw palmetto, look for capsules that contain an 85 to 90 percent concentration of liposterolic extracts. An effective dosage would be 320 milligrams daily.

Do not purchase supplements that list as their prime ingredients only saw palmetto berries or powder; these supplements may boast a higher milligram content per capsule, but they contain less, or none, of the active liposterolic extracts. Always be sure that the liposterolic amount is listed on the label.

Some people take saw palmetto as an infusion (usually 1 to 3 cups daily), as an extract (30 to 60 drops mixed in water or juice daily), or as a tincture (1 to 3 teaspoons three times daily). These methods are *not* recommended, however, because they may not provide the same beneficial liposterolic extracts found in the capsule form.

Possible side effects. Saw palmetto is generally considered a safe herb. Still, men who are taking prescription medicines for the prostate, or testosterone-blocking drugs, should consult a health care professional before taking saw palmetto.

Note. Men who are having a PSA test should alert the doctor that they are taking saw palmetto—or, if possible, should discontinue taking it a week or more prior to testing; saw palmetto slightly decreases PSA readings.

African Pygeum

African pygeum is a plant substance derived from the bark of the African plum evergreen tree. It is used extensively in Europe and is becoming well known in the United States as a treatment for prostate disorders, but not prostate cancer. Well-controlled studies have confirmed the benefits of this herbal medicine.

African pygeum contains phytosterols, pentacyclic triterpenoids, and linear alcohols—three substances that are known to do the following:

- Phytosterols reduce inflammation in the prostate by influencing the activity of prostaglandins. Prostaglandins can help reduce inflammation, but in some cases actually provoke it. For this reason, experts distinguish between good and bad prostaglandins, and phytosterols appear to block the effects of the bad kind.
- Pentacyclic triterpenoids fight inflammation in the prostate; they also inhibit the action of enzymes that cause edema (swelling caused by water buildup) within the prostate gland.
- Linear alcohols lower cholesterol levels; cholesterol is considered one factor in prostate enlargement. It should be noted that there are now drugs available that are much more effective in lowering cholesterol.

African pygeum is considered a first-line treatment for non-malignant prostate disease in Europe, Asia, Africa, and India, according to the June 2000 issue of the journal *Urological Research*. In a number of trials, patients with BPH and/or prostatitis were compared before and after treatment with African pygeum. The following results were observed:

- In the first trial, 80 percent of patients with BPH showed significant improvement, including the alleviation of most or all of their symptoms.
- In the second trial, nearly half of the men suffering from prostatitis improved; positive results were also seen in cases of dysuria (painful or difficult urination).
- The third trial showed clinical improvement in a majority of men with BPH and prostatitis; the best results, however, were seen in men whose symptoms were not severe prior to starting therapy.
- In the fourth trial, men whose mean age was seventy and who were considered good candidates for surgical treatment of BPH experienced clinical improvement after taking an African pygeum preparation for sixty days.

Among the many symptoms of BPH or prostatitis that responded well to pygeum were dysuria (painful or difficult urination), nocturia (excessive urination at night), frequency (passing water excessively), perineal heaviness (a feeling of pain or tenderness in and around the perineum), and residual urine (incomplete urination; dribbling after going to the bathroom). While African pygeum appears to relieve these symptoms of prostate dysfunction, as yet no studies have examined the role this herb may play in the prevention or treatment of prostate cancer. It should also be remembered that there are other mainstream remedies for BPH that work quite well; there are no trials comparing the effectiveness of African pygeum to standard mainstream medicines.

How to take it. In most of the trials listed above, African pygeum was taken at a dose of 200 milligrams daily. Look for a product containing 14 percent triterpenes, including beta-sitosterol and 0.5 percent n-docosanol. In some cases, patients experienced improvement in sixty days, but in others results were seen only after four months of treatment. If you combine pygeum sterols with other herbs listed in this chapter, a daily dosage of 50 to 100 milligrams is considered adequate.

Side effects. No significant side effects were noted in the trials that have been conducted. As with any other natural medicine, however, always follow the prescribed dosages, and be aware of any unusual changes or sensations that may arise. In addition, remember that herbal remedies have not been through the very rigorous testing process that new drugs are subjected to in the United States. Therefore, it is impossible for physicians or patients to be very knowledgeable about side effects or drug interactions. Also remember the PC-SPES experience. In some cases, the contents listed on the bottle do not accurately reflect all of the ingredients in the pills.

Stinging Nettle

Stinging nettle *(Urtica dioica)* is well known for the "sting" its leaves can cause when they brush against the skin. Herbalists use nettle for a variety of conditions, including asthma, infections, hair loss, and, of course, prostate disorders.

Nettle extracts contain a rich assortment of important nutrients, including iron, potassium, sulfur, magnesium, calcium, chlorophyll, and vitamins A and C. Nettle is also known to act as a diuretic (stimulant of urine flow) and an anti-inflammatory. These actions may explain nettle's possible positive effects on

BPH, prostatitis, and urinary retention. There has been less reported research on stinging nettle than saw palmetto or African pygeum.

• Stinging nettle was found to have "biologically relevant effects on human prostate cells," according to laboratory tests done at Philipps-Universitäät in Marburg, Germany, and reported in the journal *Planta Medica,* February 2000.

• An evaluation of literature on the use of herbs in the treatment of BPH concluded that stinging nettle has been found effective in the treatment of BPH, as reported in the *Annals of Pharmacotherapy,* September 2002. The study recommended that additional research be conducted on herbs for possible side effects, standardization of extracts, and concomitant use of mainstream and traditional medicine.

How to take it. Nettle is best taken in capsule form, either in combination with other herbs or on its own. When taking nettle, use only standardized extracts that contain at least 2.5 milligrams of plant silica per capsule (this is considered the most active constituent of the plant). The recommended dosage is 250 milligrams one to three times daily.

Side effects. Stinging nettle is considered a safe herb. If you prepare your own decoctions or infusions from dried leaves or powders, wear gloves to avoid a stinging sensation. Less is known about the effectiveness of this herb; if you have concerns about side effects, choose another, better-researched treatment.

NUTRITIONAL SUPPLEMENTS

As you may already suspect, eating a balanced diet may not be enough to protect your prostate from disease or to reverse prostate problems once they have started. For this reason, I often recommend that my patients take therapeutic doses of certain vitamins and minerals that may help in the treatment and prevention of prostate disease.

The April 2003 issue of the medical journal *Clinica Chimica Acta* concluded that many dietary micronutrients have been found to have "significant and complex" effects on prostate cancer cell proliferation and differentiation. The study authors also recommended additional studies to help design drugs and diet for men with prostate cancer. While awaiting additional research, it is my opinion that there is sufficient evidence to justify taking some of the nutritional supplements discussed in this chapter. However, it is important to remember that these micronutrients are not to be used as a *treatment* for prostate cancer, especially when taken alone.

Taking Supplements

Almost all supplements should be taken with a meal or up to twenty or thirty minutes before or after meals. Your body will absorb the nutrients better when taken with a meal. For example, vitamin E is not absorbed unless it is taken with food or a small amount of fat. In addition, supplements are less likely to cause stomach upset when taken with food.

Dividing your dosages (taking half in the morning and half at night, for example) will allow your body to tolerate the supplement better, if you're prone to nausea, and it will allow the supplement to remain in your bloodstream at a more steady rate over a twenty-four-hour period.

Understanding Dose Equivalents

Natural medicines for the prostate are commonly measured in grams (g), milligrams (mg), or micrograms (mcg). International units (IU) are also used.

Micrograms are the smallest measurement used when describing nutrients, followed by milligrams, and then grams. Technically speaking, one microgram is one one-thousandth of a milligram, and one milligram is one one-thousandth of a gram.

Milligrams are typically used to measure the water-soluble vitamins B and C, and for minerals such as zinc and calcium. Sometimes micrograms are used (such as when describing folic acid and selenium). International units are used to describe the oil-soluble vitamins A, D, and E.

The following chart shows the relationship between the different dosage measurements:

1,000 micrograms (1,000 mcg) = 1 milligram (1 mg)
1,000 milligrams (1,000 mg) = 1 gram (1 g)
3 milligrams (3 mg) = 5,000 international units (5,000 IU)

Zinc

Zinc is considered an important natural substance for the prostate. Zinc levels may be lowered by diarrhea, kidney disease, cirrhosis of the liver, diabetes, or the consumption of fiber, which causes zinc to be excreted through the intestinal tract. In addition, zinc levels can be disrupted by excessive perspiration and the consumption of mineralized hard water.

It appears that the cancerous prostate contains lower-than-normal levels of zinc. Clinically controlled studies have established zinc's usefulness in the treatment of benign prostate disease, but not prostate cancer. In an early study conducted in 1976, researchers found that zinc was able to reduce the symptoms associated with BPH; they also discovered a parallel between zinc deficiencies in older men and a greater risk for prostate disease. These findings have been replicated in other studies over the years.

In a more recent study, researchers found that zinc reduces prostate enlargement and can actually inhibit 5-alpha reductase, the enzyme necessary for converting testosterone to DHT. Zinc accumulates in the prostate; high levels of it inhibit the growth of prostate cancer cells in cell cultures.

Good Food Sources. Zinc can be found in a number of foods, including the following:

Source	Zinc Amount (mg per 3.5-ounce serving)
Oysters	150
Pumpkin seeds	8
Pecans	5
Brazil nuts	4
Split peas	4
Almonds	3
Lima beans	3
Oats	3
Peanuts	3
Rye	3
Walnuts	3
Whole wheat	3
Buckwheat	2
Green peas	2
Hazelnuts	2

Recommended dosages. For healthy men over age forty, 15 to 30 milligrams of zinc once daily is recommended. This dosage can be temporarily increased to 90 to 120 milligrams daily for a period of one month if you've been diagnosed with BPH or prostatitis. The dosage can then be scaled down to 60 milligrams daily after symptoms begin to improve. Many health food store prostate remedies contain 30 milligrams of zinc.

In order for zinc to be broken down in the intestinal tract, a chemical known as picolinic acid must be present. As a man ages, his level of picolinic acid decreases, making zinc absorption more difficult. To overcome this problem, men who are middle age or older should take either zinc picolinate or zinc citrate; both these forms of zinc are more readily absorbed by the small intestine, even when picolinic acid levels are low.

Side effects. Zinc can be toxic when taken in doses exceeding 200 milligrams daily for an extended period of time (several months or longer). Signs of toxicity include vomiting, stomach irritation, and mouth, tongue, and throat discomfort. The suggested therapeutic dose range of 90 to 120 milligrams for one month is not considered toxic, provided the following suggestions are carefully observed:

- Chelated forms of zinc (zinc picolinate or zinc citrate) tend to be absorbed better than other forms.
- Men suffering from viral infections such as a cold or influenza should take lower doses of zinc (no higher than 60 milligrams).
- Men with an impaired immune system (caused by a low white blood cell count, AIDS, bone marrow suppression from chemotherapy, or the like) should not take supplemental zinc.

Note. Although it does appear that prostate cancer cells have lower levels of zinc than normal cells, this does not imply that more zinc is helpful. For example, it could be the case that zinc is less able to enter prostate cells because of some characteristic related to the cell. It's also possible that prostate cancer cells are deficient in taking up zinc.

B Vitamins

The B vitamins—vitamins B_1, B_2, B_3, B_6, B_{12}, and folic acid—are said to bolster the immune system. In addition, vitamin B_6 supports the absorption of zinc, which is known to promote prostate health.

You can eat a well-balanced diet and still experience low levels of vitamin B_6. For example, certain antibiotics (which you may be taking for a prostate infection) and diuretics (which you may be taking for the treatment of edema or high blood pressure) can deplete your body of B vitamins; antidepressants can also increase the body's need for vitamin B_6.

While studies have not explicitly showed that vitamin B_6 improves prostate health or helps prevent prostate cancer, it might be a useful companion to zinc supplementation because it helps the body absorb and utilize the zinc.

Good Food Sources. Foods rich in vitamin B_6 include:

Source	B_6 Amount (mg per 3.5-ounce serving)
Brewer's yeast	3
Sunflower seeds	1
Wheat germ	1
Soybeans	0.8
Walnuts	0.7
Lentils	0.6
Lima beans	0.6

Source	B_6 Amount
	(mg per 3.5-ounce serving)
Black-eyed peas	0.6
Navy beans	0.6
Brown rice	0.6
Hazelnuts	0.5
Garbanzo beans	0.5
Pinto beans	0.5
Bananas	0.5
Avocados	0.4
Whole wheat flour	0.3
Chestnuts	0.3
Kale	0.3
Spinach	0.3
Sweet peppers	0.3
Potatoes	0.3

Recommended dosages. Take 100 milligrams of vitamin B_6 or a B-vitamin complex (which includes all of the B vitamins) daily for one month, and then 50 milligrams daily thereafter.

Caution. Taking vitamin B_6 in doses exceeding 200 milligrams daily for several months can result in nervous system toxicity. If you have any history of neurological disease, consult a physician before taking B_6.

B Vitamins by Any Other Name

Don't be confused by the different names for B vitamins:

- Vitamin B_1 is thiamin.
- Vitamin B_2 is riboflavin.

- Vitamin B_3 is niacin and niacinamide or inositol hexaniacinate (no-flush niacin).
- Vitamin B_5 is pantothenic acid or pantethine.
- Vitamin B_6 is pyridoxine.
- Vitamin B_{12} is cobalamin.
- Other B vitamins include folic acid (or folate), biotin, choline, inositol, and PABA (para-aminobenzoic acid).

The B-vitamin group is commonly known as B-complex vitamins, multiple B vitamins, stress vitamins, B-50 vitamins (for 50-milligram doses), and B-100 vitamins (100-milligram doses).

Essential Fatty Acids

Every lining cell in the body needs essential fatty acids; they are essential for building cell membranes and creating steroid hormones and bile acids. Essential fatty acids (EFAs), also known as omega-3 fatty acids, play a role in maintaining prostate health. These long-chain fatty acids contain two primary ingredients: eicosapentaenoic acid (EPA) and docosahexaenoic acid (DHA). EFAs are found in oil-rich fish such as sardines, salmon, mackerel, and herring.

In the body, the EFAs are converted into chemical substances known as prostaglandins, which act as chemical messengers that can help reduce inflammation. In addition, EFAs help transport and metabolize cholesterol and triglycerides, support brain function, maintain cell membranes, increase the metabolic rate, and improve oxygen uptake. Prostaglandins also theoretically slow the growth of cancer cells and enhance immune function. Unfortunately, about 80 percent of the

American population is believed to be deficient in omega-3 fatty acids.

Clinical trials have suggested that EFAs may have some value in the treatment of prostate disease. For example, a study conducted at the Lee Foundation for Nutritional Research in Milwaukee found that EFA therapy helped relieve symptoms of BPH. EFAs might be considered as an important adjunct in the treatment of prostate disorders. Consider the evidence:

• The results of epidemiologic and animal studies support the role of a low-fat diet supplemented with the omega-3 fatty acids in fish oil in preventing and slowing the spread of prostate cancer, as reported in the August 2001 issue of the journal *Urology.*

• According to the June 2001 issue of the British journal *Lancet,* a thirty-year follow-up study of 6,272 Swedish men found that those who ate no fish had a two- to threefold higher frequency of prostate cancer than those who ate moderate or high amounts of fish.

• The December 1999 issue of the British journal *Cancer* found that a man's risk of developing prostate cancer was reduced when he consumed essential fatty acids. The study was based on a population-controlled New Zealand study of 317 prostate cancer cases from 1996 to 1997.

Good food sources. Essential fatty acids are found in vegetable oils (flaxseed or linseed oils), soybeans, anchovies, catfish, herring, freshwater trout, mackerel, mullet, salmon, sardines, and shellfish. Generally, the fattier the fish, the higher it is in essential fatty acids.

Recommended dosages. You can receive adequate amounts of EFAs in several ways:

- Take 2 fish oil capsules with each meal (for a total of 6 capsules per day).
- Take 2 tablespoons of flaxseed or linseed oil daily. Flaxseed or linseed oils can become rancid very quickly. They should always be kept in a tightly closed bottle, refrigerated after use, and not kept more than one or two months.

Side effects. EFAs are for the most part nontoxic, but mild side effects have been reported after taking large amounts. Depending on your source of EFAs, side effects may include fishy aftertaste, diarrhea, and heartburn. Blood sugar problems and difficulties with blood clotting have also been reported in rare instances. Because of these potential side effects, people who have a family history of stroke or diabetes, as well as those on blood-thinning medications (including aspirin), should check with a doctor before taking EFAs.

Vitamin E

In addition to its antioxidant and free-radical-fighting properties, vitamin E may also improve immune system function. Natural vitamin E is more effective than synthetic versions because the body can absorb natural vitamin E twice as well as the synthetic versions.

Vitamin E is lost in heat or freezing, and when exposed to the air. Frying and processing foods, bleaching flours, and cooking all remove much of the vitamin E in whole foods. Consuming unsaturated fats actually depletes vitamin E, increasing the body's demand for it.

Vitamin E may have a protective effect against prostate cancer. Ongoing studies indicate that the effects are increased when vitamin E is taken with selenium (discussed below).

Consider the evidence: In a Finnish trial, twenty-nine thousand male smokers, age fifty to sixty-nine, were randomly assigned to receive either synthetic vitamin E (50 IU), beta-carotene (20 milligrams), both, or a placebo every day for five to eight years. The men in the vitamin E group had 32 percent lower risk of prostate cancer and a 41 percent lower risk of dying from prostate cancer within two years of beginning the trial.

Good food sources. Wheat germ, safflower oil, soybeans, uncooked green peas, spinach, asparagus, kale, cucumber, butter, and egg yolk are all high in vitamin E.

Recommended dosages. Take 400 IU of vitamin E daily in the form of natural d-alpha tocopherol.

Side effects. Some people experience a temporary increase in blood pressure after taking vitamin E supplements. If you suffer from high blood pressure, consult your physician before taking vitamin E. Your doctor will probably suggest taking 100 IU of vitamin E daily and gradually working your way up to the higher dosage while periodically checking your blood pressure.

Selenium

Selenium is a trace mineral needed by the body in very small quantities. This mineral is also known for its powerful antioxidant and anticancer effects. Specifically, selenium increases the levels of glutathione peroxidase, a substance that assists in blocking free radicals in the body. In addition, selenium enhances the effects of vitamin E.

Researchers have learned that in certain areas of the world where the level of selenium in the soil is low, there is a higher risk of many diseases, including heart disease and cancer. In the United States, where the selenium level in the soil varies from region to region depending on rainfall, there is a relationship between selenium level and disease. The level of selenium in the soil affects the level of selenium found in the foods grown in that soil. As a general rule, the more rain that falls in an area, the less selenium in the soil. The soil in the central areas of the United States contains the highest levels of selenium, while the Pacific Northwest, some eastern states, and Florida contain the least.

• As reported in the 2003 *British Journal of Urology,* men who consumed 200 micrograms of selenium daily saw a "significant protective effect" on the incidence of prostate cancer.

• The 1996 issue of the *Journal of the American Medical Association* found that selenium can have a dramatic impact on the incidence of various cancers. In a double-blind, placebo-controlled cancer prevention study done at the University of Arizona, the researchers tried to determine if selenium could reduce the risk of skin cancer recurrence. Men and women were recruited from seven dermatology clinics located in low-selenium regions of the United States. The candidates took 200 micrograms of selenium daily in the form of a high-selenium brewer's yeast tablet. The average length of time in the study for each participant was four and a half years. The selenium supplement increased participants' natural level by nearly 70 percent without any significant side effects. Although selenium had no effect on preventing skin cancer, it did cause a 63 percent decline in prostate cancer, as well as a 37 percent decrease in overall incidence of cancer, a 46 percent decrease in lung cancer, and a 58 percent decrease in colorectal cancer.

Good food sources. Brewer's yeast, wheat germ, liver, butter, fish, lamb, whole grains, nuts, molasses, Brazil nuts, brown rice, scallops, lobster, shrimp, clams, crab, and oysters are all good sources of selenium.

Recommended dosages. Take 150 to 250 micrograms of selenium daily.

Side effects. Selenium can be toxic in doses higher than 300 micrograms.

Ongoing Research

The National Cancer Institute recently began a thirty-six-thousand-patient study comparing selenium, vitamin E, and a combination of the two with a placebo or control. The main goal of the study is to see if one supplement, the other, or both together actually help prevent prostate cancer. The results of this landmark study will not be available for a decade.

Vitamin C

Antioxidant vitamins and minerals may play an important role in the management of prostate problems by helping detoxify toxic chemicals and free radicals in the body. Antioxidants also strengthen the immune system and regulate harmful stress hormones. Although vitamin C may increase the activity of the body's natural killer cells, which protect the body from cancer cells, there is little evidence that it can treat prostate cancer. It is not known if it can be a preventive agent.

Good food sources. Vitamin C is found in a number of foods:

Source	Vitamin C Amount
	(mg per 3.5-ounce serving)
Red chili peppers	375
Guavas	250
Red sweet peppers	200
Kale	175
Parsley	175
Collard greens	150
Turnip greens	140
Green sweet peppers	125
Broccoli	115
Brussels sprouts	100
Watercress	75
Cauliflower	75
Red cabbage	60
Strawberries	60
Papayas	55
Spinach	50
Oranges/orange juice	50
Lemon juice	45
Grapefruit	40
Mangoes	35
Asparagus	35
Cantaloupes	35
Green onions	30

Recommended dosages. Recommended dosages are 500 to 1,000 milligrams daily in the form of ascorbic acid tablets or capsules. This amount can be taken in two or three divided doses.

Side effects. Excess vitamin C is excreted in the urine. Side effects such as gas and diarrhea usually occur after bowel tolerance has been reached.

Lycopene

Lycopene is one of hundreds of carotenoids, or natural pigments, found in nature. The carotenoids in tomatoes make them red; they are also thought to help prevent some diseases, including cancer. In fact, laboratory studies have found lycopene to be one of the strongest antioxidants in nature. The lycopene level in cooked tomatoes is even higher than in raw tomatoes; the heat releases lycopene from the food's specific storage area and makes it more available to the body. Lycopene may not only function as an antioxidant, but also inhibit cancer cell growth by interfering with growth factor receptor signals.

Lycopene is stored in a few areas of the body, including the prostate, testicles, adrenal glands, and liver. Studies have found that men who eat more tomato sauce have lower levels of prostate cancer. Consider the evidence:

• Men who consume two to four servings of tomato sauce per week have 35 percent fewer cases of prostate cancer and 50 percent fewer cases of advanced prostate cancer, according to the November 2002 issue of *Experimental Biology and Medicine.*

• Dietary intake of lycopene from tomatoes and tomato products was associated with a decreased risk of prostate cancer, according to a study discussed in the November 2002 issue of *Experimental Biology and Medicine.* Blood and tissue lycopene levels were inversely related to the risk of prostate cancer.

• The same journal reported a randomized placebo-controlled study of thirty-two patients with local prostate cancer who ate tomato sauce (equal to 30 milligrams of lycopene per day) for three weeks before undergoing prostatectomy. Researchers found signs of lycopene uptake in the prostate tissue and a reduction in DNA damage among the men who consumed lycopene. In addition, they had a 17 percent reduction in PSA scores.

• Another study reported in the journal compared men who consumed tomato oleoresin extract with 30 milligrams of lycopene to those who took no supplements or lycopene. The former group had smaller tumors, better differentiation, and less involvement of the cancer outside the prostate.

• The February 2002 issue of *Urology Clinics of North America* concluded that it is reasonable to consume five servings of tomato products per week as part of an overall healthy diet and to reduce prostate risk, as well as the risk of other cancers.

• Some studies on lycopene have been inconclusive. The March 2002 issue of the *Journal of the National Cancer Institute* found that the association of tomato product consumption with lower risk of prostate cancer may not show up in every study because the magnitude of this association is moderate enough that it could be missed in a small study.

Good food sources. Good sources of lycopene include:

Source	Lycopene (mg per 100-gram serving)
Tomato powder	100–125
Dried tomato in oil	50
Canned pizza sauce	13
Ketchup	10–13
Tomato soup	8
Tomato sauce	6
Tomato paste	5–150
Tomato juice	5–12

Source	Lycopene (mg per 100-gram serving)
Fresh guava	3
Cooked tomatoes	4
Guava juice	3
Raw pink grapefruit	3
Watermelon	2–7
Papaya	2–5
Tomatoes, fresh	1–4
Dried apricot	1
Fresh apricot	less than 0.01

Recommended dosages. Eat tomatoes and tomato products three times a week. Little research has been performed on lycopene supplements, and if you decide to take lycopene as a supplement I would take more than 30 milligrams a day. In certain situations, antioxidants can also act as pro-oxidants—substances that actually encourage oxidative damage. Lycopene supplements have not been tested thoroughly at this time and may be a pro-oxidant in terms of prostate cancer. A recent study done on mice with human prostate cancers found that mice on lycopene supplements experienced a greater increase in their prostate cancer rates than another group of mice that was given a placebo.

Side effects. There are no known side effects to lycopene.

In addition to the use of supplements, the foods you eat can have a dramatic impact on your prostate cancer risk profile. The following chapter, The Healthy Prostate Diet, provides tips on eating to prevent and treat prostate disease.

————— ◦◦◦ —————

Chapter 10

The Healthy Prostate Diet:
Eating to Prevent and Treat
Prostate Cancer

Occasionally, prostate cancer lets its presence be known, rapidly spreading from the prostate to the bone and beyond. More commonly, the disease lies silent, harmlessly inactive as the years go by. In fact, many men live into old age without knowing that a non-life-threatening form of cancer may be growing inside their prostate glands.

Ironically, some of the most compelling evidence about prostate cancer comes not from research on men with the disease but from the autopsy room. Autopsy studies of men throughout the world have found that by age eighty, well over 50 percent of all men of every race and culture have prostate cancer. The great majority are latent or incidental cancers— tumors so small that they did not threaten the man's health, much less cause his demise. Most of these cancers were never diagnosed, and the men never knew that they had any kind of prostate problems.

One fascinating paradox of prostate cancer is that Asian men have the same level of latent cancer as men in the United States, but 90 percent less clinically apparent prostate cancer. In fact, the clinical rates of prostate cancer in China are the lowest in the world at 2.8 per 100,000 people, compared to 100 per 100,000 for Caucasians in America; that means a man is thirty-six times more likely to develop prostate cancer in the United States than in China.

This gaping difference in cancer rates is not just a reflection of genetics, but also a result of environmental factors. We know this because when men from Asia migrate to America, their prostate cancer rates increase. Actually, the biggest increase in prostate cancer is among the children and grandchildren of the immigrants, who are more likely to adopt all Western lifestyle changes, including the Western diet.

In trying to understand why Asian men living in the West have higher rates of prostate cancer, much attention has been give to the role of diet. Certainly, other factors may play a role, but some researchers suggest that overall, approximately one-third of all cancers could be avoided by dietary changes alone.

Which are the offending foods? The most likely culprits are meat and dairy products, which are higher in fat (especially saturated fat) than foods in the traditional Asian diet. The Asian diet also has a greater reliance on soy and fish for sources of protein. As a general rule, as people shift to a Western diet, they eat fewer whole grains and cereals and more animal products. They consume more saturated fats and fewer fruits and vegetables than they would in a traditional Asian diet. A number of prostate cancer researchers believe these kinds of differences in nutrition explain the differences in global distributions of the disease.

I believe that diet does play a role in the risk of acquiring prostate cancer. This is good news, because you have the power to change your diet. Furthermore, many of the foods that help protect against prostate cancer also have many general health benefits, including reducing your risk of cardiovascular disease, controlling your weight, and lowering your risk of developing other cancers. I would caution that we don't yet understand how diet affects prostate cancer risk. For example, it might be that there are herbs in Asia commonly added to foods that are unavailable here but that can reduce prostate cancer risk.

THE HEALTHY PROSTATE DIET

In simple terms, a diet rich in saturated animal fats and refined carbohydrates is likely to be unhealthy in the long run for many reasons. It may be that human evolution can't keep up with the dietary revolution that has brought us processed cheese food and double bacon cheeseburgers.

Eating well involves avoiding foods that promote prostate cancer on the one hand, and choosing foods that may help prevent cancer on the other. Don't expect to find a single magic food that will ensure prostate health. Most research confirms what you've undoubtedly heard many times before: The best way to prevent prostate cancer—as well as many other health problems—is to eat lots of fruits and vegetables, limit your consumption of red meat, restrict your overall caloric intake to maintain your optimal weight, and get regular exercise. The formula is simple, but the reality is that it is remarkably difficult for the average American to live by these basic guidelines. And even this is not a panacea for prevention; I have had numerous patients with aggressive prostate cancer who've lived a very healthy lifestyle.

DIETARY FAT

Food studies are notoriously difficult to conduct and analyze. If there is a link between prostate cancer and red meat, we must ask: Is the cancer caused by the meat itself? By the way the food is prepared? By hormones, antibiotics, and other substances that have been added to the meat? Or by the other dietary choices a man might make, because men who eat lots of red meat tend to eat fewer fruits, vegetables, and other healthier foods?

Despite the difficulties in collecting data, the research seems to show that eating animal fats, primarily red meat, is associated with increased risk of prostate cancer. For example, a study of health professionals identified a positive association between the consumption of red meat, total fat, and animal fat and the risk of prostate cancer. A follow-up study with the same men found that a high-fat diet appeared to be associated with advanced cancer, not with localized, presumably slower-growing cancer. Another study of men in Hawaii found that the risk of prostate cancer increased with the consumption of beef and animal fat. In yet another study, men who ate five or more servings of red meat each week had a 79 percent higher risk of developing prostate cancer than those men who ate less.

Researchers do not know whether the health problems stem from the fat itself or from the hormones, antibiotics, and chemicals trapped in the fat. For this reason, I recommend that you consider consuming organic or antibiotic-free meat and poultry, if you choose to include these foods in your diet. Organic meat and poultry do not necessarily have less fat, but should have fewer chemicals and contaminants.

Some researchers believe that fat stimulates the release of testosterone; both Caucasian and African American men who reduced their daily fat intake from 40 percent to 30 percent found that levels of testosterone decreased. There is controversy, however, regarding the long-term effects of testosterone on risk of prostate cancer.

To make matters more complicated, it must be noted that there are "good" fats as well as "bad" fats. For instance, fats found in fish may slow or inhibit the growth of prostate cancer cells. (Taking essential fatty acids to inhibit prostate cancer is discussed in chapter 9.)

The population studies I have discussed to this point focus mostly on the risk of getting prostate cancer, and to a lesser degree the risk of acquiring a more aggressive prostate cancer. Of course, there is also great interest in the role diet might play in men who have already been diagnosed with the disease. The question all my patients want answered is whether it is possible to slow the growth of prostate cancer during any phase of the illness with changes in diet.

Unfortunately, little is known about how dietary changes can alter the progression of prostate cancer. However tempting, it can be problematic to extrapolate the results of studies that focus on prevention into strategies for cancer treatment. A group of researchers I work with has conducted a small pilot study, in which we detected a very modest positive effect on slowing prostate cancer with soy supplements. Many more studies need to be done, however, before we can say with confidence that there is any role for diet in treating prostate cancer. Nonetheless, I counsel my patients that a diet low in saturated animal fats might be a good thing for them in any case. My patients, as men, are at a great risk for heart attack and stroke, despite having the diagnosis of prostate cancer; in fact, many will die of these diseases.

Although studies on the role of diet in altering the progression of prostate cancer in patients are lacking, animal studies have also shown that dietary fat may accelerate the rate at which cells proliferate and spread beyond the prostate. In an experiment done at Memorial Sloan-Kettering, human prostate tumors were grown in animals until they could be felt. Some of these animals were then put on a low-fat diet, while others were placed on a high-fat diet. The animals that consumed only about 20 percent of their calories from fat experienced a reduction in tumor size, while those on a higher-fat diet did not.

Scientists have found that the fatty acid linoleic acid (which is found in corn oil, safflower oil, soybean oil, and other polyunsaturated fats) can encourage the growth of prostate cancer cells in cell cultures. Linoleic acid is considered a potential promoter of tumor metastasis.

The bottom line. If possible, structure your diet so that less than 20 percent of your calories come from fat sources, of which no more than 10 percent should be saturated fat. When cutting back on fat, restrict your levels of saturated and hydrogenated fat first, then limit fat from other sources. Don't try to cut out all fat; you need some for overall health. Switch from vegetable oil to olive oil or canola oil for cooking. You may want to work with a dietician or nutritionist to design a balanced diet plan.

Know Your Fats

It can be difficult to keep track of which fats are to be avoided, and which are okay to consume in moderation. Here, in brief, is a rundown to help you when you're strolling down the aisles of the grocery stores.

Bad Fats

- *Saturated fat.* They are found in red meats, duck, chicken skin, palm oil, coconut oil, and dairy products.
- *Polyunsaturated fats.* They are found in vegetable oils (corn oil, sunflower oil, safflower oil, and other cooking oils), nuts and seeds, fish oils, and margarine. These oils are highly unstable, more prone to oxidation, and more capable of forming dangerous free radicals. Alpha-linolenic acid is a polyunsaturated fat found in red meat, margarine, and mayonnaise; it may contribute to prostate cancer.
- *Trans fats or hydrogenated vegetable oils.* Hydrogenation is the process of adding hydrogen to an unsaturated fat to make it solid. These are fats that have been processed so that they will remain solid at room temperature. They are known to contribute to arteriosclerosis and may cause oxidative damage to tissues, which can contribute to the formation of prostate and other cancers. Common sources of hydrogenated fat include Crisco, nondairy creams, harder margarines, and whipped toppings, as well as cakes, doughnuts, cookies, and other packaged snack foods.

Acceptable Fats

- *Omega-3 fatty acids.* These chains of fatty acids are found in fish oils, and they may help prevent cancer, as well as cardiovascular disease. (For more information on omega-3 fatty acids, see chapter 9.)
- *Monounsaturated fats.* These plant-based fats, such as olive oil and canola oil, are not linked to prostate cancer. Monounsaturated fats are also found in nuts, pork, oatmeal, and peanut oil. These are considered the healthiest fats.

How Much Fat Is Too Much?

In order to limit your fat intake to 20 percent of your total daily calories, you will need to know how many grams of fat you will be permitted each day. The following chart can be used as a general guide:

Average daily calories	Total daily fat grams at 30% calories from fat	Total daily fat grams at 25% calories from fat	Total daily fat grams at 20% calories from fat
1,400	47	39	31
1,600	53	45	36
1,800	60	50	40
2,000	67	56	44
2,200	73	61	49
2,400	80	67	53
2,600	87	72	58

Good Sources of Healthy Fats

Consuming omega-3 fatty acids can help inhibit the growth of prostate cancer tumors. The following foods should be included as part of a balanced diet.

Fish	Fat (grams/100 grams fish)	Omega-3 fatty acids (grams/100 grams fish)
Mackerel	13.9	2.5
Herring	9–13.9	1.6
Salmon	10.4	1.4
Bluefish	6.5	1.4
Sardines	15.5	1.4
Swordfish	2.1	1.4

Fish	Fat (grams/100 grams fish)	Omega-3 fatty acids (grams/100 grams fish)
Striped bass	2.3	0.8
Rainbow trout	3.4	0.5
Tuna	2.5	0.5
Halibut	2.3	0.4
Atlantic cod	0.7	0.3
Ocean perch	1.6	0.2

SOY

Soy is an excellent source of plant protein; it is also a powerful phytoestrogen (a plant that contains a natural source of estrogen). To make soy even more alluring, it contains cancer-fighting compounds known as isoflavonoids or isoflavones. People from countries that consume large amount of soy and other phytoestrogens typically have low rates of cancer, especially prostate and breast cancer.

The isoflavonoids in soy have multiple effects. The phytoestrogens may slightly reduce levels of testosterone. Eunuchs, men who have no testes and therefore very low levels of testosterone, are said to never get prostate cancer. Isoflavonoids also modestly inhibit some of the receptors on the cancer cells, which slows the proliferation of the cancer cells.

Unfortunately, there is recent evidence from work I am doing that there may be a negative effect to soy. In one study of postmenopausal women, soy was found to raise the levels of insulin-like growth factor 1 (a cousin of the hormone insulin). Higher levels of this hormone have been linked to an increased prostate cancer risk.

In my experience with my patients, I have seen a modest reduction in testosterone levels in men who consume soy. It is possible that soy has both positive and negative effects; life is always yin and yang.

The bottom line. Strive to consume a few servings of soy per week. If you are so motivated, you can include up to 40 grams of soy protein in your diet per day, but build up to this amount slowly. Soybeans can cause intestinal gas, so begin with 10 grams of soy protein and increase your dosage every few days to give your digestive system a chance to adjust to the high concentration of soluble fiber.

Sources of Soy

In the past few years, soy has gone mainstream. You can find a wide range of soy-based foods in most grocery stores. Those products not available from your corner grocer may be available from Asian markets or from health food stores.

- Edamame. These young soybeans can be steamed over boiling water. They are available in pods, shelled, canned, or frozen.
- Miso and miso soup. Miso is a thick paste made with soybeans, salt, and a fermenting agent. It is often mixed with rice or barley. There are three types: Hacho (which contains only soybeans), Kome (soybeans and rice), and Mugi (soybeans and barley).
- Natto. This is a fermented form of cooked soybeans; it is often used as a spread or in soups. There are those who believe fermented soy might have superior cancer-fighting properties.
- Okara. The pulp left after soy milk is strained, okara is used in granola, cookies, and vegetarian burgers.
- Soybeans. These are the basic bean from which soy products derive. They can be boiled or steamed.

- Soybean lecithin. This compound is made from soybean oil; it is often used in baked foods, candy, and chocolate coatings.
- Soy cheese. This cheese is formed with isolated soy protein; it is lactose- and cholesterol-free.
- Soy flour. This form of flour is a form of soy protein with very little starch. It should be stored in the refrigerator or freezer for freshness.
- Soy milk. This is the basis of tofu, soy yogurt, and soy cheese. It can be substituted for regular milk. It is available in plain, vanilla, chocolate, carob, and strawberry; it is sold in low-fat and nonfat versions. It is lactose-free.
- Soy nuts. They are an excellent nut substitute; they can be added to cookies or brownies in place of nuts.
- Soy oil. It does not have the same health benefits as other soy products, but it is a good source of omega-3 fatty acids.
- Soy protein powder. This is similar to soy flour, except the soybeans are cooked and then ground. Protein powder is finer than flour and has a less "beany" taste.
- Soy sauce. This form of soy has very few plant estrogens; commercial products are often filled with sugar, caramel coloring, and monosodium glutamate, a food additive. This is not a good source of soy.
- Soy yogurt. Yogurt made with soy milk is lactose- and cholesterol-free.
- Tempeh. This processed soy is similar in texture to blue cheese; it can have a mushroomlike flavor. It is sometimes used as a substitute for beef in soups, chili, and casseroles.
- Textured vegetable protein. This product, also known as texturized soy protein, can be used as a substitute for hamburger. It is similar in texture to ground beef, without cholesterol.

- Tofu. Also known as bean curd, tofu is used in a wide range of dishes. It comes in several forms:

   Firm tofu is pressed so there is less moisture.

   Soft tofu is soft but solid.

   Silken tofu has a custardlike texture.

   Smoked tofu is tofu precooked in soy sauce, then smoked.

   Dried tofu has been freeze-dried; boil it in water before use.

   Frozen tofu is a bit chewy compared to the soft version.

   As a general rule, firm and soft tofu are used for cooking, and silken is used for blending. Always check for freshness on the label. Tofu should be stored in the refrigerator.

In my own experience as a man born and raised in the Midwest, the taste and especially the texture of tofu take some getting used to. Still, soy has very positive properties; for example, it easily takes up the flavor of herbs and accompanying foods. When prepared well, tofu has become one of my favorite dishes, not only in Chinese restaurants but also at home.

Good and Good for You, Too

1 cup nonfat soy milk

2 tablespoons soy protein powder

1 tablespoon orange juice concentrate

½ medium banana, cut in pieces

½ cup strawberries

Place all the ingredients in a blender and process until smooth. You may substitute other fruits in season, if you wish. Enjoy!

LYCOPENES

According to the Harvard Men's Health Study, men who ate diets high in cooked tomatoes, which contain lycopenes, developed prostate cancer less often than those who did not consume lycopene-rich foods. For additional information on lycopene and a table listing foods containing lycopenes, see chapter 9.

The bottom line. Strive to consume cooked tomatoes and tomato sauces three or more times per week. Although the results of studies are preliminary, lycopenes available commercially as supplements may even have the affect of slowing an established prostate cancer, in addition to assisting in prevention of the disease.

CALCIUM

Calcium-rich dairy products have a reputation as healthy, wholesome foods, but this may not be true when it comes to prostate cancer. The Health Professionals Follow-up Study at Harvard University showed that men who consumed large amounts of calcium increased their risk of developing more aggressive, more advanced types of prostate cancer. Specifically, men who consumed more than 2,000 milligrams of calcium daily were three times more likely to develop advanced cancer than men who consumed less than 500 milligrams daily.

It seems that calcium interferes with the tumor-fighting

effect of vitamin D. Normally the kidneys convert vitamin D into 1,25 dihydroxy vitamin D, which seems to help keep cells well differentiated—they keep their shapes and grow in an orderly fashion. But the kidneys' ability to metabolize vitamin D depends on the amount of calcium in the bloodstream. When calcium levels are high, the body produces less 1,25 dihydroxy vitamin D. In other words, the calcium seems to block the formation of the cancer-fighting form of vitamin D.

Vitamin D is very important because prostate cells contain vitamin D receptors. When vitamin D attaches to these receptors, normal cells may be less capable of becoming cancerous, and even the growth rate of cancerous cells may slow. For example, preliminary research indicates that when patients were given 1,25 dihydroxy vitamin D, it took up to five times longer for PSA levels to double than it did in the control group.

An important source of vitamin D is sunlight. Researchers at the University of North Carolina noted that more men died of prostate cancer in the northern United States than in the southern part, perhaps because they are exposed to less sunshine in the North. The vitamin D factor may also help to explain why African American men are more prone to developing prostate cancer: African American men have more melanin in their skin than people of other races, and melanin blocks the body's ability to create vitamin D.

It appears that eating fructose (the sugar in fruit) can help engage calcium so that it doesn't alter the formation of vitamin D. Specifically, the phosphorus in fruit binds with the calcium, preventing it from altering the vitamin D balance. In fact, a study done at Harvard found that high fructose intake was associated with a reduced risk of prostate cancer.

The bottom line. Be careful about taking too much calcium. Certainly, calcium plays a role in keeping bones strong, but there may be other, more effective ways of preventing osteoporosis. Researchers are not sure, but it may be possible to counteract some of the negative effects of higher calcium intake with vitamin D. However, people should be careful even with vitamin D intake; too much can be harmful. Strive to consume five or more servings of fruits and vegetables daily. To stimulate the production of vitamin D, walk outdoors for ten to fifteen minutes two or three times a week. Most multivitamins contain about 400 IU of vitamin D.

GREEN TEA

Green tea is one of the most popular beverages in Asia, and it may help prevent both cardiovascular disease and some forms of cancer, including prostate cancer. Black tea is the type of tea most often consumed in the United States.

Black and green—as well as oolong—teas come from the same plant. The differences among the teas depend on how the leaves are processed. Green tea leaves are lightly steamed but not fermented; oolong tea leaves are partially fermented; black tea leaves are completely fermented.

During fermentation, the leaves undergo the process of oxidation, and the polyphenols (such as flavonoids or catechins in green tea) become less active. Green tea contains about 30 to 40 percent catechins (the active ingredient), while black tea contains only 5 to 10 percent; oolong tea falls in the middle. Catechins have been credited with cancer-fighting properties.

Epigallocatechin-3 gallate (EGCG) is another polyphenol that has anticancer properties against prostate cancer cells in petri dishes. One cup of green tea contains between 100 and 200 milligrams of EGCG, much more than most foods and beverages. In the laboratory, EGCG has also been shown to inhibit an enzyme known as urokinase, which may be needed for cancer growth.

As many tea drinkers know, the beverage contains caffeine. One cup of black tea contains about 35 milligrams of caffeine (about one-third the amount of caffeine in coffee), and green tea contains less than that. If you have trouble with jitteriness, high blood pressure, or irregular heartbeats when you consume caffeine, look for decaffeinated versions of both green and black tea.

The bottom line. Tea is a diuretic, so it will cause you to urinate more often. Drink plenty of additional water to compensate for any loss of water. I do not recommend the use of green tea supplements; they have not been adequately tested. It is not clear that the green tea sold in mainstream grocery stores has as much of the active ingredients as green tea sold in Chinese groceries.

Note. Green tea contains a significant amount of vitamin K, which helps the blood clot; if you are taking an anticoagulant, talk to your doctor before drinking green tea on a regular basis.

GENERAL EATING GUIDELINES

In addition to the specific food recommendations above, consider the following dietary guidelines for men concerned about prostate health:

- Avoid processed sugars and overly sweet foods. There is some evidence that excess sugar can lead to the manufacture of harmful prostaglandins, chemicals that stimulate inflammation in the prostate.
- Avoid foods containing saturated or processed fats; these include lard, palm oil, and hydrogenated or partially hydrogenated oils.

- Avoid processed cheeses, luncheon meats, and enriched, bleached, and refined foods (cakes, breads, pies, and so on).
- Eat at least two to four helpings weekly of zinc- and essential-fatty-acid-rich foods, including shellfish, cooked oysters, herring, salmon, sardines, whole fish, peas, and carrots.
- Eat at least two to four helpings weekly of soy-based foods, including soybeans, soy milk, and organic peanuts.
- Eat four or five portions per week of tomatoes and tomato-based foods, such as tomato sauce, stewed or cooked tomatoes, tomato soup, et cetera.
- Avoid fried, sautéed, charcoal-broiled, smoked, creamed, buttered, or browned foods. Instead, choose roasted, braised, steamed, baked, or poached foods. (Barbecued foods might be more healthy if you wrap them in aluminum foil during cooking; this prevents juices from dropping onto coals and forming benzoapyrenes and other potent carcinogens. Marinating foods before cooking may also cut down on some harmful compounds.)
- Eat a variety of fruits and vegetables in order to take advantage of the many different cancer-fighting compounds they contain. If you consume only two or three favorites, you will miss out on the healing effects of other produce.
- Consider organic foods. They typically cost from 15 to as much as 50 percent more than nonorganic foods, but they minimize the exposure to chemicals and additives. Note that in order to earn the U.S. Department of Agriculture's new organic seal, a product must contain at least 95 percent organic ingredients. Products containing 70

to 95 percent organic ingredients can say so on the label, but they can't display the seal.

In addition to improving your diet, there are other steps you or your loved ones may want to take to prevent prostate cancer; they will be discussed in the following chapter.

Chapter 11

Brothers and Sons:
Steps Your Loved Ones Can Take to
Prevent Prostate Cancer

Prostate cancer triggers a series of worries that flow like ripples from a pebble dropped into a pool of water. The diagnosis of prostate cancer is the initial splash, forcing a man to consider his own mortality. The next wave of worries involves the impact his cancer will have on his family and loved ones. And the subsequent ripple of anxiety is for a man's sons and brothers—the male blood relatives who may themselves be at greater risk of developing prostate cancer.

Men with prostate cancer want to do everything possible to protect their loved ones from the disease. They want to know: Why does one man develop disease, while another remains healthy? What role does heredity play? What risk factors can a man control? While not every case of prostate cancer can be prevented, there are some steps a man can take to reduce his chances of developing the disease.

THE ROLE OF HEREDITY

Some men carry one or more genes that leave them more vulnerable to prostate cancer. This is not to say that cancer is inevitable; rather, these men stand a greater risk of developing the disease. These men, identified by their family history, should be monitored closely. To assess your inherited risk, look to your family tree. You are at greater risk of developing prostate cancer if a close family member has had the disease at any age. Here are some estimates of risk based on family history. Of course, because of the multiple causes for prostate cancer, these are only estimates.

- If no one in your family has had prostate cancer, your lifetime risk of developing prostate cancer is 8 percent or one in twelve.
- If your father had prostate cancer that was not diagnosed until after age sixty, your lifetime risk of developing prostate cancer is 12 percent or one in eight.
- If your father had prostate cancer that was diagnosed before age sixty, your lifetime risk of developing prostate cancer is 20 percent or one in five.
- If your brother developed prostate cancer after age sixty, your lifetime risk of developing prostate cancer is 15 percent or one in seven.
- If your brother developed prostate cancer before age sixty, your lifetime risk of developing prostate cancer is 25 percent or one in four.
- If you have two affected first-degree male relatives (father or brothers) or maternal grandfather or uncle or paternal grandfather, at any age, your lifetime risk of developing prostate cancer is 30 percent or one in three.
- If you have three or more affected male relatives, your

lifetime risk of developing prostate cancer is 50 percent or one in two.

You can't change your genes, so you need to be aware of your risk factors.

TALKING ABOUT PROSTATE CANCER

Men need to become more comfortable talking about prostate cancer. As a society, we are a bit less tight-lipped about it than we once were, but too many men remain hesitant to discuss this form of cancer. Some men are shy about talking about a sex organ; others don't want to worry other family members about their health. Many men can learn from the example set by Betty Ford in the 1970s, when she spoke openly about her experience with breast cancer. Her openness no doubt saved many lives by encouraging women to share information about the illness.

I often sit down with a man to take a family medical history, and he has no idea how many family members may have had cancer. Sometimes there is a vague memory that an uncle may have had some sort of prostate surgery, but was the procedure for BHP or cancer?

Prostate cancer, like other malignancies, is a family disease; when a man has prostate cancer, it has an impact on his spouse and children as well. Though many men want to shield their families from knowledge about the cancer, family members have a right to know and understand your disease. I find that the families fare better when most of the aspects of this cancer are out on the table, allowing everyone to talk about it and ask questions. I encourage men to invite their spouses to office visits. Often this process can bring families closer together, helping all members reevaluate their lives and focus on what they believe to be important in life.

While I support openness, be cautious when discussing prostate cancer with friends. They will tell you about other people they know who have had prostate cancer, even though Uncle Charlie's experience with cancer may be very different from your own. Prostate cancer is a highly variable disease, and however well intentioned your friends may be, quite often their input is confusing or even annoying.

When discussing the cancer with your immediate family, try to bring the group together so that you can tell them at one time. You can avoid retelling your story repeatedly, and you can foster a balanced family dynamic without favoritism.

Reinforce with your family the idea that life is filled with ups and downs; this episode is no doubt a down, but it is not an automatic death sentence. You have no need to make acute changes in your life. Don't cancel your plans to go to Florida next summer or sell your vacation spot in the mountains. You are beginning the process of cancer management, and whether the journey is short or long, you will go through it together.

Take time to initiate dialogue with your family, both to minimize the stigma associated with disease and to talk about cancer prevention. Knowledge can be powerful, and knowledge of the family's medical history may help save the lives of your brothers and sons.

PROTECTING YOUR LOVED ONES

If you have prostate cancer, you may have particular concern about the health of your brothers and sons. While you cannot alter their genetic inheritance, you can encourage these men in your life to take the following steps:

Screening. Prostate cancer screening—PSA tests and regular digital rectal exams—is controversial because it is not clear that it results in decreased cancer death rates. However, screening is more likely to be useful in high-risk populations, so I recommend screening for men with any increased heredity risk. (My screening recommendations for the general population are summarized in chapter 2.) In addition to detecting cancer at earlier stages, screening helps many men manage their anxiety about the disease by allowing them to take concrete steps to monitor it.

Herbs and nutritional supplements. Although we do not yet have prevention trial evidence showing a reduction in prostate cancer, I recommend vitamin E and selenium supplements and a diet rich in lycopene to men with a hereditary predisposition to prostate cancer. When used responsibly, these nutrients will do no harm, and there is convincing research to indicate that they may help prevent or delay some cancers in some men. For more information on herbs and nutritional supplements, including dosing information, see chapter 9.

Diet. A balanced, plant-based, low-fat diet rich in fruits and vegetables is good for you, whether or not you have a greater genetic risk of developing prostate cancer. Keep in mind that cardiovascular disease kills more men than prostate cancer, and eating right can help prevent heart disease as well. For additional information about eating for a healthy prostate, see chapter 10.

Exercise. There is some evidence that regular exercise may help prevent the onset of cancer, including prostate cancer. Exercise reduces stress, raises lean body mass, and changes the metabolism of testosterone. Recent studies have shown that obesity is related to a higher death rate for all forms of cancer. In addition, regular exercise is part of an overall healthy lifestyle.

These steps may not prevent prostate cancer, but they may, in fact, delay its onset.

What I'm Doing to Avoid Prostate Cancer

I preach prevention, but do I take my own advice? I do my best. I have no family history of prostate cancer, and I'm in the over-fifty age group. I do the following to prevent prostate cancer for myself:

- Every day, I take:
    - 400 international units of vitamin E.
    - 200 micrograms of selenium.
    - 50 milligrams of a B-complex vitamin with additional vitamin C.
    - A multivitamin.
- Three or four times a week, I exercise (running, swimming, biking).
- I follow a low-fat diet (no saturated animal fats), and I try to eat lots of tomato sauces (rich in lycopenes) and cruciferous vegetables (high in antioxidants).
- I have my PSA level tested each year.

Once a man learns he has prostate cancer, he often finds a great deal of empathy and advice from other men who are battling the disease as well. The following chapter, You Are Not Alone, offers advice on finding the right support group for men with prostate cancer.

Chapter 12

You Are Not Alone: Finding the Right Prostate Cancer Support Group and Talking About Your Cancer

Alan Greenspan, Norman Schwarzkopf, Bob Dole, Rudy Giuliani, Bill Bixby, Joe Torre, Arnold Palmer, Telly Savalas—we recognize these men as military heroes, athletes, politicians, and actors. We know a great deal about their professional accomplishments—and also their private lives, including intimate facts about their medical history: All of these men have had prostate cancer.

In the past ten years or so, prostate cancer has come out of the closet—at least partway. Prostate cancer can now be a topic of polite conversation; it can be discussed in mixed company without speaking in whispers and hushed tones. Information about prostate cancer is reported widely by the media, and as a result men are better informed about the disease than they were just a few years ago.

That said, a simple truth remains: Men may talk openly about prostate cancer in general terms, but for some good reasons they remain squeamish about discussing the matter when it involves their personal health. Face it, incontinence, sexual dysfunction, impotence, and other complications of prostate cancer aren't popular topics in the locker room or on the golf course.

While men may not feel comfortable confiding in their friends and colleagues, a growing number of men are sharing their experiences with other men in prostate cancer survivor groups. These groups offer the kind of information and coping skills that only other cancer survivors can provide. They help men understand their disease, gather information about doctors and treatment options, and, most important, gain emotional support during a difficult and confusing experience.

Support groups can be very effective at providing reassurance to men who have been recently diagnosed with prostate cancer. During the initial phase of adjustment, most men focus on classic questions: *Will I live? Will I remain potent? Will I have pain? Will I be able to urinate in the same way?* These are life-altering questions. At some point during an open discussion, it will become obvious that everyone else is struggling with these same questions. Prostate cancer support groups can offer intimate, firsthand experiences and assurances that can be far more powerful than even the best-intentioned doctor.

Research shows that people who participate in support groups may actually experience higher survival rates. A study reported in the August 15, 1995, issue of the journal *Cancer* found that social support appeared to be associated with longer survival among women with localized or regional-stage breast cancer. There is every reason to believe the same findings would apply to men with prostate cancer. Yet even if support groups don't help men live longer, for the right people, they certainly help men live better.

On a personal level, I have seen patients almost transformed by their experience in a support group. One man who was very depressed and angry about his diagnosis altered his whole outlook after an evening in which he saw that there were many men just like him, and several much worse off. Still, I know that support groups aren't for everyone. Some men are more comfortable keeping their medical histories and feelings within their immediate family and doctor's office. There is nothing at all wrong with this approach.

Prostate cancer support groups also help educate patients about their treatment options. As mentioned earlier, many doctors believe they hold a comprehensive discussion of the illness and treatment options with each patient, while the vast majority of prostate cancer patients leave the doctor's office burdened with unanswered questions. In the study reported in the September 1997 issue of the journal *Urology* (and mentioned in chapter 3) almost 100 percent of the physicians questioned stated that they "always" discussed treatment options with their patients, but only one-fifth of the patients questioned reported having these discussions. Clearly doctors and patients need to improve communication so that men receive all the information they need to consider their treatment options.

In the same study, it was also found that while both doctors and patients believed that physicians were an excellent source of educational support, they also agreed that doctors did not provide adequate emotional support. Men with prostate cancer have emotional and educational needs that probably can't be completely met by most physicians and their staffs. Some doctors fail to appreciate the important service provided by support groups. I believe that prostate cancer groups provide a critical network of support to men with the disease, as well as to their families.

In many cases, support groups may offer more benefits to

family members, especially partners of affected men, than to patients themselves. In our local group, we have sessions for the wives alone, in which they have the opportunity to discuss issues related to sexuality and the possibility of loss. Sometimes the spouse attends the meetings of the prostate cancer support group, and the patient stays home. This can be a fine strategy as long as all participants are able to get what they need in a way that feels comfortable and is convenient. As I've said before, prostate cancer is a family disease. Everyone in the family is affected by the anxiety of the diagnosis, and couples are affected by the obvious intrusions into sexuality. Good support groups will address the needs of all, without mandating a specific approach or necessity for everyone to share everything.

PROSTATE CANCER'S SILVER LINING

For men with prostate cancer—and their families—life is divided into two parts: life before cancer and life after it. My patients repeatedly tell me that time stops and they feel emotionally numb as soon as they hear the word *cancer*. They can remember with extreme accuracy everything about that precise moment, from the clothes they were wearing to the color of the carpet and the dust on the telephone. From that moment forward, nothing is ever quite the same.

It also bears noting that there is a silver lining to prostate cancer: It can help a man live more consciously. Cancer forces most men to reassess their lives and to appreciate that life, for each of us, is finite. One patient who comes to mind is a man in his forties who had been overwhelmingly dedicated to gaining status in his career. He made great compromises in his personal life to achieve his professional goals. After his diagnosis, however, he reassessed his life and made different choices, which made him a better husband, a better father, and a better man. Ironically, he became more productive and creative at work. In the end, he viewed the cancer as a blessing; the disease helped him refocus his life. This process of personal evolution is quite common among men with prostate cancer, as well as other life-threatening conditions.

Even in the heartbreaking cases when a man does not survive, the cancer often helps him live his last years with greater focus on matters of importance. Early in my career, I had a patient who was estranged from his son. His cancer was quite advanced, and it was clear that he was going to die. I asked if I could contact his son. The man consented, and we found the son in Santa Fe, New Mexico. The son flew to the East Coast, and father and son were reunited and reconciled. That may not have happened if the cancer had not been detected.

Another man with young children learned he had an aggressive cancer and made dramatic shifts in his life. He had been an investment banker in the high-flying financial times. After his diagnosis, he spent more time with his children. He made it to the second-grade play. Instead of spending mornings in the office, he made peanut-butter-and-jelly sandwiches with his children and helped them get off to school. He said he wouldn't wish prostate cancer on anyone, but the five years he had left with his family were much richer and more meaningful than he thinks they would have been without the disease. Cancer often reminds us of our own mortality, and that can be a blessing, especially when it reminds us to cherish the moment and live in the present.

FINDING THE RIGHT SUPPORT GROUP

When you participate in a support group, you may want to share intimate facts about your life and health. Alternatively, you may not feel comfortable opening up to strangers in every type of support setting. You can, however, increase the odds of finding a good match by choosing the right type of group.

Support groups can be organized in a number of different ways. Some are just for patients with prostate cancer and their family members; others are open to anyone affected by any type of cancer. The different focus of the group should help meet the particular needs of the men involved. For example, men newly diagnosed with localized cancer will have different concerns than those shared by men with recurrent cancer or advanced cancer.

Support groups may also have either open or closed membership. *Open membership* refers to groups in which a man may come and go within the group freely. He may come to two or three meetings, skip five or six, then return to the group at another point. This means the membership will change with each meeting. Some people find it more difficult to develop intimate relationships and to build trust in these groups, but they are effective for many men.

In a closed group, members register and commit to attend as many meetings as they can. The group is usually limited in number and meets for a fixed time period. In these groups, men have a greater opportunity to develop trust and intimacy. Given the challenges of balancing other commitments and time demands, however, this is not a practical choice for everyone.

ORGANIZATIONS OF INTEREST

The following organizations can help you locate a prostate cancer support group in your area. You should also ask your doctor. Many physicians who have been practicing for a long time in the community are aware of local support groups.

American Cancer Society

1599 Clifton Road Northeast
Atlanta, GA 30329
404-320-3333 or 808-ACS-2345
www.cancer.org

This national organization sponsors a prostate cancer support group known as Man to Man. In addition, the group provides comprehensive information about prostate cancer, makes referrals to treatment centers, and provides free publications.

Prostate Cancer Support Group Network

c/o American Foundation for Urologic Disease
1000 Corporate Blvd.
Suite 410
Linthicum, MD 21090
410-689-3990 or 800-828-7866
www.afud.org

PCSN, affiliated with the American Foundation for Urologic Disease, provides services for several support groups, self-help organizations, and their members.

Us Too! International, Inc.

5003 Fairview Avenue
Downers Grove, IL 60515
800-80-US-TOO or 630-795-1002
www.ustoo.org

This international nonprofit organization operates support groups for men with prostate cancer and their families. Us Too! meetings are free and open to family members, friends, and health care workers interested in prostate disease.

HOW TO TALK ABOUT YOUR CANCER

It's easy to share good news. In fact, it can be hard to contain your joy when you tell someone that you just won the lottery, earned a big promotion, or bought a new sports car. Sharing bad news, especially news about your health, is much more difficult.

Most of my patients choose to keep their diagnosis private, at least for the first few weeks. While it is important to have the support of friends and colleagues, you should share information at your own pace, and then only with those you trust.

As any man who has gone through the experience knows, the first few weeks after diagnosis are a blur. This is a time for you to focus on taking care of yourself. Sleep late if you want to, go for a long walk, take extra time at the gym, or eat an extra dessert. Do whatever you need to do to feel like you're nurturing yourself.

Dealing with a difficult medical situation can be especially challenging for men because they tend to try to control the situations in their lives. A man may be at the top of his professional and personal life, but he may feel completely inadequate and powerless when handling this disease. You need to accept that having prostate cancer is a new experience for you, and one that may generate debilitating anxiety and feelings of helplessness. The anxiety will dissipate when you realize that treatment is available and that in the coming weeks you will make progress at coping with this situation.

When I speak to men immediately after their diagnosis, they believe they are forever changed. For the vast majority of men, however, life will someday return to what they considered normal. Prostate cancer will no longer be the first thing they think about in the morning when they wake and the last thing they think about at night before sleep. They will once again obsess about their 401(k) accounts and curse the traffic during their morning commute. It may be weeks or months—sometimes longer—but the petty concerns of life will someday regain their importance.

For most men, the period of severe anxiety lasts until the treatment phase is complete. During the first few weeks, men are uncomfortable and on edge during office visits and treatments. After a few weeks, most men grow more relaxed and regain some level of comfort with themselves. For most patients, good news will put their minds at ease, although most men feel anxious when they undergo subsequent PSA tests because they fear a recurrence of the disease.

Talking with your spouse or partner. When a man is diagnosed with prostate cancer, family roles may change. A man may need to rest more than he once did. He may be unable to do certain chores. He may be emotionally withdrawn or emotionally available, depending on his frame of mind.

I have seen prostate cancer make a bad marriage into a good marriage and a good marriage even stronger. I have also seen it weaken a marriage because the couple cannot communicate their needs and expectations to one another. In each situation, both the man and his partner may benefit by being able to discuss their feelings in a safe and supportive environment. This can sometimes be accomplished in the doctor's office, but time there is limited. Again, support groups for both the man suffering from prostate cancer and for family members can help the family work through these challenges.

I don't see it as much as I used to, but I continue to encounter patients who do not want to tell their wives about the disease. This is often counterproductive, given the issues of erectile dysfunction. In many cases, they want to protect them from the truth, though this can be a form of denial. I encourage those patients who are able to share the information with their partners so that they can work together as a couple to manage the illness and get the support they need individually and as a family.

Accept that at times, you and your partner will feel out of step with one another. One of you may feel optimistic about the future at a time when the other feels frightened. One of you may become deeply involved in work or outside commitments, while the other focuses exclusively on the cancer and its treatment. The key to managing these differences is open communication; each person is using different coping strategies to work through the situation. By understanding what your partner is feeling, you can respect your differences and find ways to work together.

Of course, there is no "right" way to deal with the stress and anxiety of a cancer diagnosis and treatment. There is nothing inherently wrong with going inside yourself for a while. Sometimes it is only during quiet times that a patient can find a way to communicate with a higher power and find strength and acceptance.

Talking with other relatives. It is best to become educated about the disease before discussing it with relatives other than your spouse. It is important to know that a diagnosis of prostate cancer is not a death sentence. You may find yourself reassuring your friends and family members that you will be okay. You will probably have to educate them about the disease.

Before discussing the cancer with friends and family, think through your feelings and your expectations of them. People react very differently to this kind of information, so you should be ready to accept a wide range of reactions. Trusted friends may seem awkward and uncomfortable; they may withdraw. Others may try to become too involved in your illness in such a way that you feel your privacy is being violated.

Feel free to set the boundaries that make you feel comfortable. If possible, tell friends what they can do to help. Try to be as direct and open as you can. You will help other people cope in this way.

A major problem with talking to friends about prostate cancer is that they will try to help in ways that are not always appreciated. Specifically, they may mention a new treatment they heard about in the news or that their cousin had that they claim was a breakthrough. Often the treatment in question was for a different stage of prostate cancer. Also, many treatments featured in newscasts that are presented as on the horizon may actually not be available for years, if ever. In this way, well-intentioned friends can induce needless anxiety.

Talking with employers and co-workers. I believe that most men should be judicious about discussing their disease at the workplace. The gossip grapevine exists at every office, and once word of your illness is out, you will be a source of gossip. You can't put the genie back in the bottle and recapture your privacy after it has been lost, so I encourage my patients to keep the matter to themselves until they feel confident that they will be comfortable with questions from co-workers.

You need to think through the dynamics at work before telling your employer about your condition. Discuss with your doctor the ways that your illness or treatment may interfere with your job performance. If you need to take time off from work for treatment, you should inform your employer, but you do not need to divulge every detail of your illness. You have certain legal protections against discrimination on the job, and you should become aware of your rights if your employer threatens your position or your health care coverage. It's always a good idea to keep detailed records of any discussions you have about your illness with your employer or workers in the benefits office.

Talking to children. However uncomfortable it may be, at some point you will need to discuss your cancer with your children. How you do so depends on the age and maturity of the children, of course. You need to be honest with your children so that they will know you aren't keeping secrets from them. They can only feel safe if they know that you are telling them the truth. Many people who try to "spare" their children from the truth end up regretting that they were not more open.

In most cases, you can't keep the information from your children, even if you try. Children will pick up on the stress and anxiety in the household, and they will glean information from conversations they overhear and from fears they may have. They may be more anxious than the situation warrants.

If possible, wait until the period of overwhelming stress and strong emotions has passed to talk to your children about prostate cancer. If you discuss the situation with them with too much fear and anxiety, your children will be unable to find reassurance in your words. The calmer you are, the less frightened the children will be.

Don't overwhelm young children with too much information. Assure them that they will receive excellent care. Explain that there are many different types of cancer and that each person's situation is different.

Though it seems unnecessary, remind your children that this is not their fault. Children naturally see their world as revolving around them; in many cases they believe that they did something to cause the cancer. Children need to be reassured that the disease has nothing to do with their behavior.

When discussing the initial diagnosis with your children, give them a basic explanation of the situation, and then give them time to digest what they have heard. Although the words you choose will depend on the age and maturity of your child, if you have early-stage localized cancer you might try words such as:

> I want you to know that I have cancer inside my body. I am lucky because it is not very big, and I have a good doctor who will help me get rid of it. I may have to go to the doctor a lot in the next few months, but you don't need to worry. I love you very much, and there will always be someone to help take care of you. You are safe and sound, and you did nothing to cause this to happen. It can be difficult to understand, so I want you to come to me and ask questions anytime you want to know more, okay?

Expect them to ask questions, but don't be discouraged if they don't right away. Children basically want to know if you will be okay. Over time, as the household activities resume, most children will feel some comfort that not everything is changing just because Dad has cancer.

Some kids may benefit from participating in their own support group for children whose parents have cancer. A support group provides a safe place for the children to discuss their feelings and frustrations. The disease and its treatment may have an impact on their entire family, children may have a wide range of feelings about the situation. Many hospitals, psychologists, and school counselors offer support groups.

HOW TO BE A GOOD FRIEND

If you want to talk with someone about his cancer—or any other serious illness—it is sometimes difficult to find the right words. Keep these tips in mind:

- Let the person with the illness take the lead. Be there to listen.
- Accept periods of silence. Try to be present without filling every pause in the conversation with nervous chatter. Sometimes the most meaningful part of a conversation happens between the words.
- Look the person in the eye. Touch the person on the arm, if that is natural to you. Smile. Affirming gestures make a difference and show the person that you care, even though he is sick.
- Don't offer advice. Most people aren't eager to hear about what you think they should do or how someone you know handled a similar illness or situation. Let the other person be the expert about his situation.
- Avoid saying "I know how you feel." It's not about you.
- If you can't keep your own emotions in check, explain this to the person you are speaking to and excuse yourself. You do not want the person with the illness to spend his energy comforting you.
- If appropriate, tell a joke, share a story, talk about something other than illness. Take cues from the person you are talking with about whether he would enjoy diversions or if he needs to speak about his illness.
- Keep up with the regular activities of your relationship. If you used to share a hobby or go out to dinner once a week, maintain these activities. Accept that the person may have less energy than he used to, but resume as many activities as the person chooses.
- Don't be a stranger. Some people avoid contact with a person with a serious illness because they don't know what to do or say. Maintain your relationship. You can ask to help with errands or chores around the house, if you think that would be easier. Some people feel more

comfortable "working" as an expression of concern rather than directly communicating.

If you are sensitive to the needs of your friend or loved one, your genuine affection will come through, even if you struggle for the right words. So the best you can to support your friend, and no doubt your efforts will be appreciated.

International Prostate Symptom Score Sheet

To assess symptoms of Benign Prostatic Hyperplasia (BPH) answer the questions with one of the following scores:

0 (not at all)
1 (less than one time in five)
2 (less than half the time)
3 (about half the time)
4 (more than half the time)
5 (almost always)

1. Incomplete emptying: Over the past month, how often have you had a sensation of not emptying your bladder completely after you finished urinating? ____
2. Frequency: Over the past month, how often have you had to urinate again less than two hours after you finished urinating? ____

3. Intermittency: Over the past month, how often have you found you stopped and started again several times when you urinated? _____

4. Urgency: Over the past month, how often have you found it difficult to postpone urination? _____

5. Weak stream: Over the past month, how often have you had a weak urinary stream? _____

6. Straining: Over the past month, how often have you had to push or strain to begin urination? _____

7. Nocturia: Over the past month, how many times did you most typically get up to urinate from the time you went to bed at night until the time you got up in the morning? _____

8. Quality of life: If you were to spend the rest of your life with your urinary condition just the way it is now, how would you feel about that? _____

    0   Delighted
    1   Pleased
    2   Mostly satisfied
    3   Mixed: about equally satisfied and dissatisfied
    4   Mostly dissatisfied
    5   Unhappy
    6   Terrible

Add your scores. The total is your International Prostate Symptom Score (IPSS).

If your total score is:
  0–7   Your symptoms are considered mild.
 8–19   Your symptoms are considered moderate.
20–35   Your symptoms are considered severe.

Appendix B

———○○○———

The Partin Tables

To use the information on these pages, find your PSA level, then scan the list for your appropriate Gleason score and clinical stage. (For clarification of the meaning of the Gleason and clinical stage scores, see chapter 4.)

If your PSA is 0–2.5 ng/ml,
  and your Gleason score is 2–4,
    and your clinical stage is T1c, there is:

- a 95 percent chance your cancer is organ confined.
- a 5 percent chance your cancer has penetrated the capsule.
- a 0 percent chance the seminal vesicles are involved.
- a 0 percent chance the lymph nodes are involved.

  and your clinical stage is T2a, there is:

- a 91 percent chance your cancer is organ confined.
- a 9 percent chance your cancer has penetrated the prostate capsule.

- a 0 percent chance your seminal vesicles are involved.
- a 0 percent chance your lymph nodes are involved.

and your clinical stage is T2b, there is:

- an 88 percent chance your cancer is organ confined.
- a 12 percent chance your cancer has penetrated the prostate capsule.
- a 0 percent chance your seminal vesicles are involved.
- a 0 percent chance your lymph nodes are involved.

and your clinical stage is T2c, there is:

- an 86 percent chance your cancer is organ confined.
- a 14 percent chance your cancer has penetrated the prostate capsule.
- a 0 percent chance your seminal vesicles are involved.
- a 0 percent chance your lymph nodes are involved.

**and your Gleason score is 5–6,
and your clinical stage is T1c, there is:**

- a 90 percent chance your cancer is organ confined.
- a 9 percent chance your cancer has penetrated the prostate capsule.
- a 0 percent chance your seminal vesicles are involved.
- a 0 percent chance your lymph nodes are involved.

and your clinical stage is T2a, there is:

- an 81 percent chance your cancer is organ confined.
- a 17 percent chance your cancer has penetrated the prostate capsule.
- a 1 percent chance your seminal vesicles are involved.
- a 0 percent chance your lymph nodes are involved.

and your clinical stage is T2b, there is:

- a 75 percent chance your cancer is organ confined.
- a 22 percent chance your cancer has penetrated the prostate capsule.
- a 2 percent chance your seminal vesicles are involved.
- a 1 percent chance your lymph nodes are involved.

and your clinical stage is T2c, there is:

- a 73 percent chance your cancer is organ confined.
- a 24 percent chance your cancer has penetrated the prostate capsule.
- a 1 percent chance your seminal vesicles are involved.
- a 1 percent chance your lymph nodes are involved.

and your Gleason score is 3 + 4 = 7, and your clinical stage is T1c, there is:

- a 79 percent chance your cancer is organ confined.
- a 17 percent chance your cancer has penetrated the prostate capsule.
- a 2 percent chance your seminal vesicles are involved.
- a 1 percent chance your lymph nodes are involved.

and your clinical stage is T2a, there is:

- a 64 percent chance your cancer is organ confined.
- a 29 percent chance your cancer has penetrated the prostate capsule.
- a 5 percent chance your seminal vesicles are involved.
- a 2 percent chance your lymph nodes are involved.

and your clinical stage is T2b, there is:

- a 54 percent chance your cancer is organ confined.
- a 35 percent chance your cancer has penetrated the prostate capsule.
- a 6 percent chance your seminal vesicles are involved.

- a 4 percent chance your lymph nodes are involved.

and your clinical stage is T2c, there is:

- a 51 percent chance your cancer is organ confined.
- a 36 percent chance your cancer has penetrated the prostate capsule.
- a 5 percent chance your seminal vesicles are involved.
- a 6 percent chance your lymph nodes are involved.

and your Gleason score is 4 + 3 = 7,
    and your clinical stage is T1c, there is:

- a 71 percent chance your cancer is organ confined.
- a 25 percent chance your cancer has penetrated the prostate capsule.
- a 2 percent chance your seminal vesicles are involved.
- a 1 percent chance your lymph nodes are involved.

and your clinical stage is T2a, there is:

- a 53 percent chance your cancer is organ confined.
- a 40 percent chance your cancer has penetrated the prostate capsule.
- a 4 percent chance your seminal vesicles are involved.
- a 3 percent chance your lymph nodes are involved.

and your clinical stage is T2b, there is:

- a 43 percent chance your cancer is organ confined.
- a 45 percent chance your cancer has penetrated the prostate capsule.
- a 5 percent chance your seminal vesicles are involved.
- a 6 percent chance your lymph nodes are involved.

and your clinical stage is T2c, there is:

- a 39 percent chance your cancer is organ confined.

- a 45 percent chance your cancer has penetrated the prostate capsule.
- a 5 percent chance your seminal vesicles are involved.
- a 9 percent chance your lymph nodes are involved.

and your Gleason score is 8–10,
and your clinical stage is T1c, there is:

- a 66 percent chance your cancer is organ confined.
- a 28 percent chance your cancer has penetrated the prostate capsule.
- a 4 percent chance your seminal vesicles are involved.
- a 1 percent chance your lymph nodes are involved.

and your clinical stage is T2a, there is:

- a 47 percent chance your cancer is organ confined.
- a 42 percent chance your cancer has penetrated the prostate capsule.
- a 7 percent chance your seminal vesicles are involved.
- a 3 percent chance your lymph nodes are involved.

and your clinical stage is T2b, there is:

- a 37 percent chance your cancer is organ confined.
- a 46 percent chance your cancer has penetrated the prostate capsule.
- a 9 percent chance your seminal vesicles are involved.
- a 6 percent chance your lymph nodes are involved.

and your clinical stage is T2c, there is:

- a 34 percent chance your cancer is organ confined.
- a 47 percent chance your cancer has penetrated the prostate capsule.
- an 8 percent chance your seminal vesicles are involved.
- a 10 percent chance your lymph nodes are involved.

If your PSA is 2.6–4.0 ng/ml,
  and your Gleason score is 2–4,
    and your clinical stage is T1c, there is:

- a 92 percent chance your cancer is organ confined.
- an 8 percent chance your cancer has penetrated the prostate capsule.
- a 0 percent chance your seminal vesicles are involved.
- a 0 percent chance your lymph nodes are involved.

  and your clinical stage is T2a, there is:

- an 85 percent chance your cancer is organ confined.
- a 15 percent chance your cancer has penetrated the prostate capsule.
- a 0 percent chance your seminal vesicles are involved.
- a 0 percent chance your lymph nodes are involved.

  and your clinical stage is T2b, there is:

- an 80 percent chance your cancer is organ confined.
- a 20 percent chance your cancer has penetrated the prostate capsule.
- a 0 percent chance your seminal vesicles are involved.
- a 0 percent chance your lymph nodes are involved.

  and your clinical stage is T2c, there is:

- a 78 percent chance your cancer is organ confined.
- a 22 percent chance your cancer has penetrated the prostate capsule.
- a 0 percent chance your seminal vesicles are involved.
- a 0 percent chance your lymph nodes are involved.

  and your Gleason score is 5–6,
    and your clinical stage is T1c, there is:

- an 84 percent chance your cancer is organ confined.
- a 15 percent chance your cancer has penetrated the prostate capsule.
- a 1 percent chance your seminal vesicles are involved.
- a 0 percent chance your lymph nodes are involved.

and your clinical stage is T2a, there is:

- a 71 percent chance your cancer is organ confined.
- a 27 percent chance your cancer has penetrated the prostate capsule.
- a 2 percent chance your seminal vesicles are involved.
- a 0 percent chance your lymph nodes are involved.

and your clinical stage is T2b, there is:

- a 63 percent chance your cancer is organ confined.
- a 34 percent chance your cancer has penetrated the prostate capsule.
- a 2 percent chance your seminal vesicles are involved.
- a 1 percent chance your lymph nodes are involved.

and your clinical stage is T2c, there is:

- a 61 percent chance your cancer is organ confined.
- a 36 percent chance your cancer has penetrated the prostate capsule.
- a 2 percent chance your seminal vesicles are involved.
- a 1 percent chance your lymph nodes are involved.

and your Gleason score is 3 + 4 = 7,
and your clinical stage is T1c, there is:

- a 68 percent chance your cancer is organ confined.
- a 27 percent chance your cancer has penetrated the prostate capsule.
- a 4 percent chance your seminal vesicles are involved.

- a 1 percent chance your lymph nodes are involved.

and your clinical stage is T2a, there is:

- a 50 percent chance your cancer is organ confined.
- a 41 percent chance your cancer has penetrated the prostate capsule.
- a 7 percent chance your seminal vesicles are involved.
- a 2 percent chance your lymph nodes are involved.

and your clinical stage is T2b, there is:

- a 41 percent chance your cancer is organ confined.
- a 47 percent chance your cancer has penetrated the prostate capsule.
- a 9 percent chance your seminal vesicles are involved.
- a 3 percent chance your lymph nodes are involved.

and your clinical stage is T2c, there is:

- a 38 percent chance your cancer is organ confined.
- a 48 percent chance your cancer has penetrated the prostate capsule.
- an 8 percent chance your seminal vesicles are involved.
- a 5 percent chance your lymph nodes are involved.

and your Gleason score is 4 + 3 = 7,
and your clinical stage is T1c, there is:

- a 58 percent chance your cancer is organ confined.
- a 37 percent chance your cancer has penetrated the prostate capsule.
- a 4 percent chance your seminal vesicles are involved.
- a 1 percent chance your lymph nodes are involved.

and your clinical stage is T2a, there is:

- a 39 percent chance your cancer is organ confined.

- a 52 percent chance your cancer has penetrated the prostate capsule.
- a 6 percent chance your seminal vesicles are involved.
- a 2 percent chance your lymph nodes are involved.

and your clinical stage is T2b, there is:

- a 30 percent chance your cancer is organ confined.
- a 57 percent chance your cancer has penetrated the prostate capsule.
- a 7 percent chance your seminal vesicles are involved.
- a 4 percent chance your lymph nodes are involved.

and your clinical stage is T2c, there is:

- a 27 percent chance your cancer is organ confined.
- a 57 percent chance your cancer has penetrated the prostate capsule.
- a 6 percent chance your seminal vesicles are involved.
- a 7 percent chance your lymph nodes are involved.

and your Gleason score is 8–10,
and your clinical stage is T1c, there is:

- a 52 percent chance your cancer is organ confined.
- a 40 percent chance your cancer has penetrated the prostate capsule.
- a 6 percent chance your seminal vesicles are involved.
- a 1 percent chance your lymph nodes are involved.

and your clinical stage is T2a, there is:

- a 33 percent chance your cancer is organ confined.
- a 53 percent chance your cancer has penetrated the prostate capsule.
- a 10 percent chance your seminal vesicles are involved.
- a 3 percent chance your lymph nodes are involved.

and your clinical stage is T2b, there is:

- a 25 percent chance your cancer is organ confined.
- a 57 percent chance your cancer has penetrated the prostate capsule.
- a 12 percent chance your seminal vesicles are involved.
- a 5 percent chance your lymph nodes are involved.

and your clinical stage is T2c, there is:

- a 23 percent chance your cancer is organ confined.
- a 57 percent chance your cancer has penetrated the prostate capsule.
- a 10 percent chance your seminal vesicles are involved.
- an 8 percent chance your lymph nodes are involved.

If your PSA is 4.1–6.0 ng/ml,
   and your Gleason score is 2–4,
      and your clinical stage is T1c, there is:

- a 90 percent chance your cancer is organ confined.
- a 10 percent chance your cancer has penetrated the prostate capsule.
- a 0 percent chance your seminal vesicles are involved.
- a 0 percent chance your lymph nodes are involved.

and your clinical stage is T2a, there is:

- an 81 percent chance your cancer is organ confined.
- a 19 percent chance your cancer has penetrated the prostate capsule.
- a 0 percent chance your seminal vesicles are involved.
- a 0 percent chance your lymph nodes are involved.

and your clinical stage is T2b, there is:

- a 75 percent chance your cancer is organ confined.

- a 25 percent chance your cancer has penetrated the prostate capsule.
- a 0 percent chance your seminal vesicles are involved.
- a 0 percent chance your lymph nodes are involved.

and your clinical stage is T2c, there is:

- a 73 percent chance your cancer is organ confined.
- a 27 percent chance your cancer has penetrated the prostate capsule.
- a 0 percent chance your seminal vesicles are involved.
- a 0 percent chance your lymph nodes are involved.

and your Gleason score is 5–6,
and your clinical stage is T1c, there is:

- an 80 percent chance your cancer is organ confined.
- a 19 percent chance your cancer has penetrated the prostate capsule.
- a 1 percent chance your seminal vesicles are involved.
- a 0 percent chance your lymph nodes are involved.

and your clinical stage is T2a, there is:

- a 66 percent chance your cancer is organ confined.
- a 32 percent chance your cancer has penetrated the prostate capsule.
- a 1 percent chance your seminal vesicles are involved.
- a 1 percent chance your lymph nodes are involved.

and your clinical stage is T2b, there is:

- a 57 percent chance your cancer is organ confined.
- a 39 percent chance your cancer has penetrated the prostate capsule.
- a 2 percent chance your seminal vesicles are involved.
- a 2 percent chance your lymph nodes are involved.

and your clinical stage is T2c, there is:

- a 55 percent chance your cancer is organ confined.
- a 40 percent chance your cancer has penetrated the prostate capsule.
- a 2 percent chance your seminal vesicles are involved.
- a 3 percent chance your lymph nodes are involved.

and your Gleason score is 3 + 4 = 7,
and your clinical stage is T1c, there is:

- a 63 percent chance your cancer is organ confined.
- a 32 percent chance your cancer has penetrated the prostate capsule.
- a 3 percent chance your seminal vesicles are involved.
- a 2 percent chance your lymph nodes are involved.

and your clinical stage is T2a, there is:

- a 44 percent chance your cancer is organ confined.
- a 46 percent chance your cancer has penetrated the prostate capsule.
- a 5 percent chance your seminal vesicles are involved.
- a 4 percent chance your lymph nodes are involved.

and your clinical stage is T2b, there is:

- a 35 percent chance your cancer is organ confined.
- a 51 percent chance your cancer has penetrated the prostate capsule.
- a 7 percent chance your seminal vesicles are involved.
- a 7 percent chance your lymph nodes are involved.

and your clinical stage is T2c, there is:

- a 31 percent chance your cancer is organ confined.

- a 50 percent chance your cancer has penetrated the prostate capsule.
- a 6 percent chance your seminal vesicles are involved.
- a 12 percent chance your lymph nodes are involved.

and your Gleason score is 4 + 3 = 7,
and your clinical stage is T1c, there is:

- a 52 percent chance your cancer is organ confined.
- a 42 percent chance your cancer has penetrated the prostate capsule.
- a 3 percent chance your seminal vesicles are involved.
- a 3 percent chance your lymph nodes are involved.

and your clinical stage is T2a, there is:

- a 33 percent chance your cancer is organ confined.
- a 56 percent chance your cancer has penetrated the prostate capsule.
- a 5 percent chance your seminal vesicles are involved.
- a 6 percent chance your lymph nodes are involved.

and your clinical stage is T2b, there is:

- a 25 percent chance your cancer is organ confined.
- a 60 percent chance your cancer has penetrated the prostate capsule.
- a 5 percent chance your seminal vesicles are involved.
- a 10 percent chance your lymph nodes are involved.

and your clinical stage is T2c, there is:

- a 21 percent chance your cancer is organ confined.
- a 57 percent chance your cancer has penetrated the prostate capsule.
- a 4 percent chance your seminal vesicles are involved.
- a 16 percent chance your lymph nodes are involved.

and your Gleason score is 8–10,
  and your clinical stage is T1c, there is:

- a 46 percent chance your cancer is organ confined.
- a 45 percent chance your cancer has penetrated the prostate capsule.
- a 5 percent chance your seminal vesicles are involved.
- a 3 percent chance your lymph nodes are involved.

  and your clinical stage is T2a, there is:

- a 28 percent chance your cancer is organ confined.
- a 58 percent chance your cancer has penetrated the prostate capsule.
- an 8 percent chance your seminal vesicles are involved.
- a 6 percent chance your lymph nodes are involved.

  and your clinical stage is T2b, there is:

- a 21 percent chance your cancer is organ confined.
- a 59 percent chance your cancer has penetrated the prostate capsule.
- a 9 percent chance your seminal vesicles are involved.
- a 10 percent chance your lymph nodes are involved.

  and your clinical stage is T2c, there is:

- an 18 percent chance your cancer is organ confined.
- a 57 percent chance your cancer has penetrated the prostate capsule.
- a 7 percent chance your seminal vesicles are involved.
- a 16 percent chance your lymph nodes are involved.

If your PSA is 6.1–10.0 ng/ml,
  and your Gleason score is 2–4,
    and your clinical stage is T1c, there is:

- an 87 percent chance your cancer is organ confined.
- a 13 percent chance your cancer has penetrated the prostate capsule.
- a 0 percent chance your seminal vesicles are involved.
- a 0 percent chance your lymph nodes are involved.

and your clinical stage is T2a, there is:

- a 76 percent chance your cancer is organ confined.
- a 24 percent chance your cancer has penetrated the prostate capsule.
- a 0 percent chance your seminal vesicles are involved.
- a 0 percent chance your lymph nodes are involved.

and your clinical stage is T2b, there is:

- a 69 percent chance your cancer is organ confined.
- a 31 percent chance your cancer has penetrated the prostate capsule.
- a 0 percent chance your seminal vesicles are involved.
- a 0 percent chance your lymph nodes are involved.

and your clinical stage is T2c, there is:

- a 67 percent chance your cancer is organ confined.
- a 33 percent chance your cancer has penetrated the prostate capsule.
- a 0 percent chance your seminal vesicles are involved.
- a 0 percent chance your lymph nodes are involved.

and your Gleason score is 5–6,
and your clinical stage is T1c, there is:

- a 75 percent chance your cancer is organ confined.
- a 23 percent chance your cancer has penetrated the prostate capsule.
- a 2 percent chance your seminal vesicles are involved.

- a 0 percent chance your lymph nodes are involved.

and your clinical stage is T2a, there is:

- a 58 percent chance your cancer is organ confined.
- a 37 percent chance your cancer has penetrated the prostate capsule.
- a 4 percent chance your seminal vesicles are involved.
- a 1 percent chance your lymph nodes are involved.

and your clinical stage is T2b, there is:

- a 49 percent chance your cancer is organ confined.
- a 44 percent chance your cancer has penetrated the prostate capsule.
- a 5 percent chance your seminal vesicles are involved.
- a 2 percent chance your lymph nodes are involved.

and your clinical stage is T2c, there is:

- a 46 percent chance your cancer is organ confined.
- a 46 percent chance your cancer has penetrated the prostate capsule.
- a 5 percent chance your seminal vesicles are involved.
- a 3 percent chance your lymph nodes are involved.

**and your Gleason score is 3 + 4 = 7,
and your clinical stage is T1c, there is:**

- a 54 percent chance your cancer is organ confined.
- a 36 percent chance your cancer has penetrated the prostate capsule.
- an 8 percent chance your seminal vesicles are involved.
- a 2 percent chance your lymph nodes are involved.

and your clinical stage is T2a, there is:

- a 35 percent chance your cancer is organ confined.

- a 49 percent chance your cancer has penetrated the prostate capsule.
- a 13 percent chance your seminal vesicles are involved.
- a 3 percent chance your lymph nodes are involved.

and your clinical stage is T2b, there is:

- a 26 percent chance your cancer is organ confined.
- a 52 percent chance your cancer has penetrated the prostate capsule.
- a 16 percent chance your seminal vesicles are involved.
- a 6 percent chance your lymph nodes are involved.

and your clinical stage is T2c, there is:

- a 24 percent chance your cancer is organ confined.
- a 52 percent chance your cancer has penetrated the prostate capsule.
- a 13 percent chance your seminal vesicles are involved.
- a 10 percent chance your lymph nodes are involved.

and your Gleason score is 4 + 3 = 7,
and your clinical stage is T1c, there is:

- a 43 percent chance your cancer is organ confined.
- a 47 percent chance your cancer has penetrated the prostate capsule.
- an 8 percent chance your seminal vesicles are involved.
- a 2 percent chance your lymph nodes are involved.

and your clinical stage is T2a, there is:

- a 25 percent chance your cancer is organ confined.
- a 58 percent chance your cancer has penetrated the prostate capsule.
- an 11 percent chance your seminal vesicles are involved.
- a 5 percent chance your lymph nodes are involved.

and your clinical stage is T2b, there is:

- a 19 percent chance your cancer is organ confined.
- a 60 percent chance your cancer has penetrated the prostate capsule.
- a 13 percent chance your seminal vesicles are involved.
- an 8 percent chance your lymph nodes are involved.

and your clinical stage is T2c, there is:

- a 16 percent chance your cancer is organ confined.
- a 58 percent chance your cancer has penetrated the prostate capsule.
- an 11 percent chance your seminal vesicles are involved.
- a 13 percent chance your lymph nodes are involved.

and your Gleason score is 8–10, and your clinical stage is T1c, there is:

- a 37 percent chance your cancer is organ confined.
- a 48 percent chance your cancer has penetrated the prostate capsule.
- a 13 percent chance your seminal vesicles are involved.
- a 3 percent chance your lymph nodes are involved.

and your clinical stage is T2a, there is:

- a 21 percent chance your cancer is organ confined.
- a 57 percent chance your cancer has penetrated the prostate capsule.
- a 17 percent chance your seminal vesicles are involved.
- a 5 percent chance your lymph nodes are involved.

and your clinical stage is T2b, there is:

- a 15 percent chance your cancer is organ confined.

- a 57 percent chance your cancer has penetrated the prostate capsule.
- a 19 percent chance your seminal vesicles are involved.
- an 8 percent chance your lymph nodes are involved.

and your clinical stage is T2c, there is:

- a 13 percent chance your cancer is organ confined.
- a 56 percent chance your cancer has penetrated the prostate capsule.
- a 16 percent chance your seminal vesicles are involved.
- a 13 percent chance your lymph nodes are involved.

If your PSA is more than 10.0 ng/ml,
  and your Gleason score is 2–4,
    and your clinical stage is T1c, there is:

- an 80 percent chance your cancer is organ confined.
- a 20 percent chance your cancer has penetrated the prostate capsule.
- a 0 percent chance your seminal vesicles are involved.
- a 0 percent chance your lymph nodes are involved.

  and your clinical stage is T2a, there is:

- a 65 percent chance your cancer is organ confined.
- a 35 percent chance your cancer has penetrated the prostate capsule.
- a 0 percent chance your seminal vesicles are involved.
- a 0 percent chance your lymph nodes are involved.

  and your clinical stage is T2b, there is:

- a 57 percent chance your cancer is organ confined.
- a 43 percent chance your cancer has penetrated the prostate capsule.

- a 0 percent chance your seminal vesicles are involved.
- a 0 percent chance your lymph nodes are involved.

and your clinical stage is T2c, there is:

- a 54 percent chance your cancer is organ confined.
- a 46 percent chance your cancer has penetrated the prostate capsule.
- a 0 percent chance your seminal vesicles are involved.
- a 0 percent chance your lymph nodes are involved.

and your Gleason score is 5–6,
and your clinical stage is T1c, there is:

- a 62 percent chance your cancer is organ confined.
- a 33 percent chance your cancer has penetrated the prostate capsule.
- a 4 percent chance your seminal vesicles are involved.
- a 2 percent chance your lymph nodes are involved.

and your clinical stage is T2a, there is:

- a 42 percent chance your cancer is organ confined.
- a 47 percent chance your cancer has penetrated the prostate capsule.
- a 6 percent chance your seminal vesicles are involved.
- a 4 percent chance your lymph nodes are involved.

and your clinical stage is T2b, there is:

- a 33 percent chance your cancer is organ confined.
- a 52 percent chance your cancer has penetrated the prostate capsule.
- an 8 percent chance your seminal vesicles are involved.
- an 8 percent chance your lymph nodes are involved.

and your clinical stage is T2c, there is:

- a 30 percent chance your cancer is organ confined.
- a 51 percent chance your cancer has penetrated the prostate capsule.
- a 6 percent chance your seminal vesicles are involved.
- a 13 percent chance your lymph nodes are involved.

and your Gleason score is 3 + 4 = 7,
  and your clinical stage is T1c, there is:

- a 37 percent chance your cancer is organ confined.
- a 43 percent chance your cancer has penetrated the prostate capsule.
- a 12 percent chance your seminal vesicles are involved.
- an 8 percent chance your lymph nodes are involved.

and your clinical stage is T2a, there is:

- a 20 percent chance your cancer is organ confined.
- a 49 percent chance your cancer has penetrated the prostate capsule.
- a 16 percent chance your seminal vesicles are involved.
- a 14 percent chance your lymph nodes are involved.

and your clinical stage is T2b, there is:

- a 14 percent chance your cancer is organ confined.
- a 47 percent chance your cancer has penetrated the prostate capsule.
- a 17 percent chance your seminal vesicles are involved.
- a 22 percent chance your lymph nodes are involved.

and your clinical stage is T2c, there is:

- an 11 percent chance your cancer is organ confined.
- a 42 percent chance your cancer has penetrated the prostate capsule.
- a 13 percent chance your seminal vesicles are involved.

- a 33 percent chance your lymph nodes are involved.

and your Gleason score is 4 + 3 = 7,
  and your clinical stage is T1c, there is:

- a 27 percent chance your cancer is organ confined.
- a 51 percent chance your cancer has penetrated the prostate capsule.
- an 11 percent chance your seminal vesicles are involved.
- a 10 percent chance your lymph nodes are involved.

and your clinical stage is T2a, there is:

- a 14 percent chance your cancer is organ confined.
- a 55 percent chance your cancer has penetrated the prostate capsule.
- a 13 percent chance your seminal vesicles are involved.
- an 18 percent chance your lymph nodes are involved.

and your clinical stage is T2b, there is:

- a 9 percent chance your cancer is organ confined.
- a 50 percent chance your cancer has penetrated the prostate capsule.
- a 13 percent chance your seminal vesicles are involved.
- a 27 percent chance your lymph nodes are involved.

and your clinical stage is T2c, there is:

- a 7 percent chance your cancer is organ confined.
- a 43 percent chance your cancer has penetrated the prostate capsule.
- a 10 percent chance your seminal vesicles are involved.
- a 38 percent chance your lymph nodes are involved.

and your Gleason score is 8–10,
  and your clinical stage is T1c, there is:

- a 22 percent chance your cancer is organ confined.
- a 50 percent chance your cancer has penetrated the prostate capsule.
- a 17 percent chance your seminal vesicles are involved.
- an 11 percent chance your lymph nodes are involved.

and your clinical stage is T2a, there is:

- an 11 percent chance your cancer is organ confined.
- a 52 percent chance your cancer has penetrated the prostate capsule.
- a 19 percent chance your seminal vesicles are involved.
- a 17 percent chance your lymph nodes are involved.

and your clinical stage is T2b, there is:

- a 7 percent chance your cancer is organ confined.
- a 46 percent chance your cancer has penetrated the prostate capsule.
- a 19 percent chance your seminal vesicles are involved.
- a 27 percent chance your lymph nodes are involved.

and your clinical stage is T2c, there is:

- a 6 percent chance your cancer is organ confined.
- a 41 percent chance your cancer has penetrated the prostate capsule.
- a 15 percent chance your seminal vesicles are involved.
- a 38 percent chance your lymph nodes are involved.

SOURCE: Partin, A. W.; Walsh, P. C.; Epstein, J. I.; and Pearson, J. D. "Contemporary Update of Prostate Cancer Staging Nomograms (Partin Tables) for the New Millennium," *Urology* 58, 2001.

Appendix C

Additional Resources

ORGANIZATIONS OF INTEREST

American Foundation for Urologic Disease
1000 Corporate Blvd.
Suite 410
Linthicum, MD 21090
410-689-3990 or 800-828-7866
www.afud.org
This nonprofit group supports the prevention and cure of prostate cancer and other urologic diseases through public education, research, and advocacy. The foundation operates a toll-free hot line and a Prostate Cancer Support Group Network that links prostate cancer support groups and survivors.

Cancer Care, Inc.
275 Seventh Avenue
New York, NY 10001
212-302-2400 or 800-813-HOPE

www.cancercare.org

This national nonprofit organization provides free professional help to patients and families through counseling, education, information, referral, and direct financial assistance.

National Association for Continence
P. O. Box 8310
Spartanburg, SC 29305-8310
800-BLADDER or 864-579-7900
www.nafc.org

The association supports public education about the causes of and treatments for incontinence.

National Cancer Institute Cancer Information Service
Public Inquiries:
Building 31, Room 10A31
31 Center Drive, MSC 2580
Bethesda, MD 20892-2580
301-435-3848 or 800-4-CANCER
TTY 800-332-8615
www.nci.nih.gov/hpage/cis.htm

This is a national clearinghouse for educational information on prostate cancer, as well as other forms of cancer. NCI sponsors the Cancer Information Service, a toll-free phone service that provides information to patients, their families, and health professionals.

Us Too! International, Inc.
5003 Fairview Avenue
Downers Grove, IL 60515
800-80-US-TOO or 630-795-1002
www.ustoo.org

This nonprofit organization operates support groups for men with prostate cancer, and for their families. Chapter meetings are free and open to family members, friends, and health care professionals interested in prostate cancer. The group also publishes a monthly newsletter.

WEB SITES OF INTEREST

www.oncolink.com

The University of Pennsylvania Cancer Center resource site provides extensive information about prostate cancer. The site includes a listing of clinical trials and an Ask the Experts section.

www.phoenix5.org

This nonprofit site is designed to help men and their companions overcome the lifestyle challenges associated with prostate cancer, including impotence.

www.prostate.com

This site provides an excellent overview of prostate cancer and prostate disease. It includes advice on treatment options; those using this site should be aware that it is sponsored by a pharmaceutical company that sells a drug used in the treatment of prostate cancer.

www.prostate-online.com

Virgil's On-line Guide to Fighting Prostate Cancer includes a posting of research findings, personal experiences, and background information. It also includes information on clinical trials.

www.prostateforum.com

The Prostate Forum is a subscription-based monthly newsletter that provides useful, reliable, timely information about prostate cancer and its treatment in easy-to-understand language.

www.prostatepointers.org/iceballs
This site includes basic information, research findings, and news reports about cryotherapy and its use in treating prostate cancer.

www.WebMD.com
A comprehensive and interactive health information service that includes information relevant to prostate cancer survivors and their families.

INTERNET BULLETIN BOARDS OF INTEREST

www.sharedexperience.com
This Web site allows you to share your experiences with cancer, including an open discussion of how side effects from treatments have changed your lifestyle. This site is also open to friends and family members of people with cancer to help them better understand how it feels to live with the disease.

www.prostatepointers.org/p2p
Physician to Patients (p2p) is a moderated list designed to allow patients to ask specific questions of qualified health care providers. Keep in mind that all advice posted from this or any other Web site should be cleared by your personal physician.

www.prostatepointers.org/iceballs
"Iceballs" is an Internet discussion group offering information and first-person accounts from men who have used cryosurgery in the treatment of prostate cancer.

Glossary

acid phosphatase/prostate acid phosphatase (PAP) An enzyme secreted by the prostate gland. Elevated levels of prostate acid phosphatase in the blood can indicate that prostate cancer cells are present. PAP testing cannot be used for cancer screening because it does not identify cancer cells until they spread beyond the prostate. It is a test that is less frequently used today.

adenocarcinoma A tumor that develops in the glandular tissue of the prostate. This is by far the most common type of prostate tumor.

adjuvant therapy A treatment that is used to supplement the primary form of therapy.

adrenal glands Glands (one located above each of the two kidneys) that produce a number of different hormones, some of which can be converted to testosterone.

alpha blockers Prescription drugs used to treat high blood pressure. They have been found to relax a circular muscle in the urethra and therefore permit more complete emptying of the bladder. Alpha blockers are therefore sometimes used in the treatment of BPH.

anal-digital rectal examination (DRE) Direct finger examination of the prostate via the rectum. This procedure should be included as part of any comprehensive physical exam.

androgens   The male hormones, including testosterone and dihydrotestosterone. These hormones are essential for the development and health of male sexual organs.

angiogenesis   The process of growing new blood vessels. Drugs known as angiogenesis inhibitors are being investigated for their ability to treat cancer by blocking the development of new blood vessels around the tumors. The cancer is not destroyed, but is not permitted to advance.

antiandrogens   Prescription drugs used to block testosterone from binding to its receptor. (Examples include Casodex, Eulexin, and Nilandron.)

BPH (benign prostatic hyperplasia)   A noncancerous enlargement of the prostate. BPH can cause urinary problems as the excessive tissue presses on the urethra. It can also result in elevated PSA levels.

BPH (benign prostatic hypertrophy)   Similar to benign prostatic hyperplasia, this condition is caused by an increase in the size of the existing cells rather than an increase in the number of cells. There is little clinical distinction between this condition and benign prostatic hyperplasia.

benign   A condition that is not cancerous.

brachytherapy   A prostate cancer treatment that involves the insertion of radioactive pellets into the prostate; this treatment is also called interstitial radiation therapy or seed therapy.

cachexia   Weight loss associated with advanced stages of cancer and other diseases.

cryotherapy   A procedure, sometimes referred to as cryosurgery, in which liquid nitrogen is used to freeze tumors within the prostate. The liquid nitrogen passes through probes inserted through the perineum and into the prostate. Cryotherapy kills both healthy and cancerous tissue.

cystitis Inflammation of the bladder, usually caused by a bacterial infection.

digital rectal examination See *anal-digital rectal examination.*

dihydrotestosterone (DHT) A hormone produced by the breakdown of the male sex hormone testosterone by the enzyme 5-alpha reductase. DHT can be found within the prostate and has been linked to an overgrowth of prostate tissue. DHT levels tend to increase in men after age fifty.

dysuria Difficult or painful urination.

erectile dysfunction Also known as impotence, this is the partial or complete inability to have or maintain an erection for sexual intercourse. Erectile dysfunction may be a side effect of prostate surgery, radiation therapy, or hormone treatment.

5-alpha reductase An enzyme required for the breakdown of testosterone into dihydrotestosterone.

Gleason score A method of classifying prostate cancer cells. The less distinctive or differentiated the cancer cells are compared to normal cells, the more aggressive the cancer. The higher the Gleason score, the more malignant the cancer. Well-differentiated patterns give a sum of 5 or 6; moderately differentiated cells are given a score of 7; and poorly differentiated cells are given an 8, 9, or 10. The Gleason score is a sum of the predominant pattern and the second most common pattern. Therefore, Gleason scores of 7 can be expressed as 3 + 4 or 4 + 3. The latter is more aggressive.

gynecomastia Enlargement or tenderness of a man's breasts or nipples. This condition is a possible side effect of some forms of hormonal therapy.

hematospermia Blood in the semen.

hematuria   Blood in the urine. Hematuria can be gross (visible to the naked eye) or microscopic (detected only with a microscope).

isoflavones   Chemicals found in foods such as beans, peas, and soy products; some studies indicate that isoflavones may help inhibit the formation of prostate cancer.

latent prostate cancer   This is a type of prostate cancer that does not threaten the life of the patient. It is also known as incidental prostate cancer.

LHRH (luteinzing hormone–releasing hormone) agonists   Drugs used to inhibit the production of testosterone from the testicles.

lymph node sampling   A procedure in which a surgeon examines abdominal lymph nodes to see if the prostate cancer has metastasized beyond the gland. The sampling is usually performed during prostate surgery.

metastasis   The medical term for cancer spreading to remote sites in the body from the primary tumor. (*Metastasize* is a verb meaning "to spread by metastasis.")

nocturia   Urination during the night.

oncologist (medical)   A physician who specializes in the treatment of cancer with drugs or hormones.

oncologist (radiation)   A physician who specializes in the treatment of cancer with different forms of radiation.

orchiectomy   The surgical removal of one or both of the testicles. In the treatment of prostate cancer, orchiectomy may be used instead of LHRH-agonists, such as lupron or goserelin.

PC-SPES   A combination of many herbs formulated to control the progress of prostate cancer. Some of the herbs are strong phytoestrogens (plant estrogens).

perineum   The region between the scrotum and the anus.

prostate   The walnut-shaped gland located directly beneath the bladder. This gland produces much of the seminal fluid.

prostatic intraepithelial neoplasia (PIN)   Irregular cells detected on a biopsy that may indicate a propensity to develop cancer in that region. If PIN cells are detected, a patient will probably be asked to have a repeat biopsy in three months to one year.

prostatic urethra   A tube that passes urine and sperm through the prostate.

prostatitis   Inflammation of the prostate, usually caused by a bacterial or nonbacterial infection.

PSA test   A blood test that measures levels of a protein known as prostate-specific antigen. Elevated PSA levels may indicate prostate cancer, though PSA scores can be raised by BPH, prostatitis, and other conditions as well.

RPP (radical perineal prostatectomy)   A surgery in which the prostate is removed through an incision in the perineum.

RRP (radical retropubic prostatectomy)   A surgery in which the prostate is removed through an incision made in the abdomen.

residual urine   Urine that remains in the bladder after a man finishes urinating.

retrograde ejaculation   A condition in which sperm passes into the bladder and is released in the urine. Some prostate procedures (such as TURP) can lead to retrograde ejaculation.

seed therapy   See *brachytherapy.*

seminal fluid   The whitish fluid released during ejaculation; the fluid contains sperm and secretions from the prostate gland.

testosterone   The male sex hormone that accounts for about 90 percent of androgens in a man's body.

TRUS-P (transrectal ultrasound of the prostate)   A medical procedure in which a probe releasing high-frequency sound waves is inserted in the rectum; the sound waves are converted into a picture of the prostate gland.

TUBD (transurethral balloon dilatation) A procedure for treating BPH in which a constricted urethra is opened using a balloonlike device.

TUIP (transurethral incision of the prostate) A surgical procedure for BPH in which the urethra is separated from the enlarged prostate tissue surrounding it.

TULIP (transurethral laser-induced prostatectomy) A surgical procedure for BPH in which swollen prostate tissue is destroyed using lasers.

TUMT (transurethral microwave thermotherapy) A surgical procedure for BPH in which swollen prostate tissue is destroyed using microwave heat.

TUNA (transurethral needle ablation of the prostate) A surgical procedure for BPH in which swollen prostate tissue is reduced using ultrasound energy discharged through needles inserted into the prostate.

TURP (transurethral resection of the prostate) A surgical procedure for BPH in which swollen prostate tissue is removed using a special tube inserted through the urethra. This is one of the most common surgical procedures used to treat BPH.

urethritis Inflammation of the urethra (the tube that carries urine from the bladder and out through the penis). Urethritis is often caused by bladder and kidney infections.

urinary incontinence The leakage of urine from the urethra.

watchful waiting An approach to managing less aggressive forms of prostate cancer in which the patient does not receive treatment but is watched and monitored to see if the disease progresses. Because prostate cancer often grows very slowly, watchful waiting is the treatment of choice for many older men.

Index

About the Authors

DR. GLENN J. BUBLEY is an associate professor of medicine at Harvard Medical School and director of Genitourinary Oncology at Beth Israel Deaconess Medical Center, a facility that takes an interdisciplinary approach to cancer treatment. Dr. Bubley is also an expert clinical researcher who investigates therapies for prostate cancer. Dr. Bubley treats prostate cancer patients and does clinical and basic research on prostate cancer treatment and prevention. Dr. Bubley is a diplomate of the American Board of Internal Medicine, subspecialty Medical Oncology; he is also an ad hoc reviewer for the medical journals *New England Journal of Medicine, Cancer Research, Cancer, Journal of Clinical Oncology,* and *Urology.* He is director of the Hershey Family Foundation for Prostate Cancer Research, and a member of the Conquer and Cure Prostate Cancer board of directors.

WINIFRED CONKLING is a medical writer based in northern Virginia. She has written more than twenty books on a variety of health topics.